ATLAS

OF

THE MOUTH

AND

ADJACENT PARTS

IN

HEALTH AND DISEASE

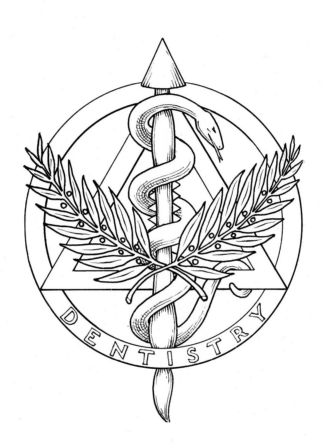

ATLAS

OF

THE MOUTH

AND

ADJACENT PARTS

IN

HEALTH AND DISEASE

Prepared by

MAURY MASSLER, D.D.S., M.S.

*Director of the Child Research Clinic, Assistant Professor of Histology and
Lecturer in Stomatology (College of Medicine)*

and

ISAAC SCHOUR, D.D.S., Ph.D., D.Sc.

Professor of Histology and Head of the Department of Histology

UNIVERSITY OF ILLINOIS, COLLEGE OF DENTISTRY

Drawings by
CARL T. LINDEN

180 Illustrations (19 in Color)

Published and Distributed by

THE BUREAU OF PUBLIC RELATIONS
COUNCIL ON DENTAL HEALTH

AMERICAN DENTAL ASSOCIATION
222 E. SUPERIOR ST., CHICAGO, ILL.

FOREWORD

THE growing interest in oral and dental health on the part of the public and the health professions has created a demand for an Atlas of the Mouth. The plates which compose this Atlas were selected primarily to illustrate those anatomic structures and physiologic conditions as well as certain pathologic conditions of the oral cavity that are of common interest to both the dentist and the physician. Because of the scope of the Atlas, no attempt was made to treat any one subject exhaustively. Sufficient attention was, however, given to the visual presentation of oral structures and relationships to provide the clinician with a sound background for diagnosis and treatment. Some of the subjects discussed are not readily available in the dental literature. A few are the result of original research. It is hoped that the study and enjoyment of these plates will stimulate the reader to seek further information.

Many of the plates are original. Others are adapted from older works and brought up to date in the light of newer knowledge. All were skillfully executed by the artist, Mr. Carl T. Linden, under the supervision of Professor Tom Jones, head of the Illustration Department of the Chicago Colleges of the University of Illinois. The illustrations were lettered by Miss Marion Mason. Most of the illustrations were originally prepared for a forthcoming text on "The Mouth and Its Diseases," by the authors.

M. M.
I. S.

CONTENTS

CONTENTS

THE ORAL CAVITY

THE oral cavity is the special province of the dentist. It contains more than teeth and gingivae. Examination of the lips, the tongue, the floor of the mouth, the buccal mucosa, the palate, the temporomandibular joint, the fauces and even the tonsils and the throat should be a routine part of the dental examination.

Recognition of early pathologic changes in the oral cavity of systemic as well as local origin is the responsibility of the dentist and a part of the dental health service.

THE ORAL CAVITY

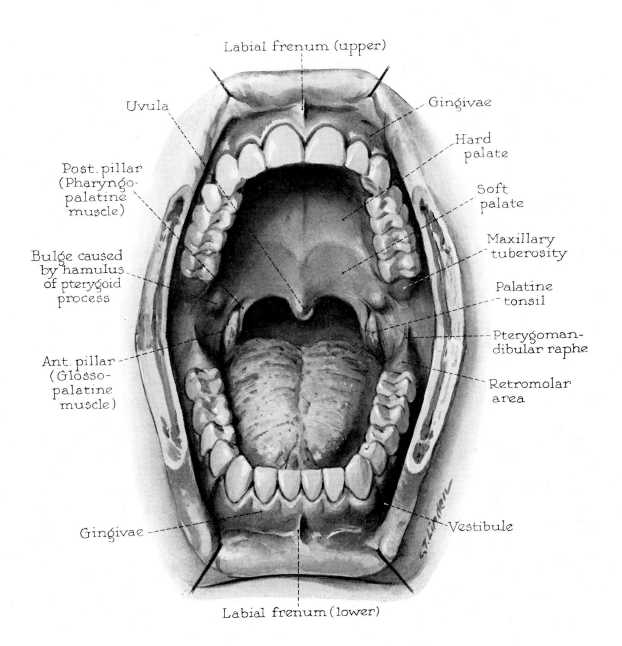

Labial frenum (upper)

Uvula

Gingivae

Hard palate

Post. pillar
(Pharyngo-
palatine
muscle)

Soft
palate

Bulge caused
by hamulus
of pterygoid
process

Maxillary
tuberosity

Palatine
tonsil

Pterygoman-
dibular raphe

Ant. pillar
(Glosso-
palatine
muscle)

Retromolar
area

Gingivae

Vestibule

Labial frenum (lower)

PLATE I.

THE PERMANENT ARCH

THE integrity of each arch depends on the normal curvilinear arrangement of the teeth, with each tooth in contact with its adjacent neighbors. A break or irregularity in the contact line, which is caused by the loss or displacement of a single tooth, or a part of a tooth, results in the imbalance of the entire arch (malocclusion). (See Plate 10.)

The teeth of opposing arches interdigitate in such a manner that the upper arch overlaps and confines the lower, and each tooth is opposed by two teeth of the other arch (except the upper third molars and lower central incisors).

ERUPTION OF THE PERMANENT TEETH

	Lower	Upper
	Age (years)	Age (years)
Central Incisors	6- 7	7- 8
Lateral Incisors	7- 8	8- 9
Cuspids	9-10	11-12
First Bicuspids	10-12	10-11
Second Bicuspids	11-12	10-12
First Molars	6- 7	6- 7
Second Molars	11-13	12-13
Third Molars	17-21	17-21

The lower teeth erupt before the corresponding upper teeth.
The teeth usually erupt earlier in girls than in boys.

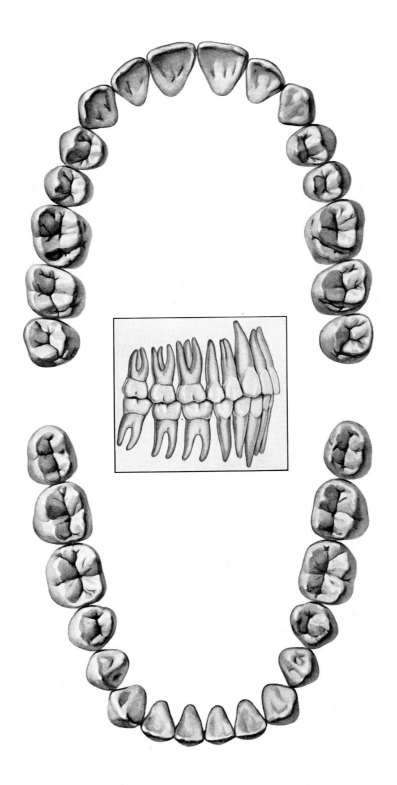

PLATE 2.

THE DECIDUOUS ARCH

THE integrity of the permanent arch depends on the care given to the deciduous teeth. Prevention of dental disease and protective dental treatment should start with the deciduous dentition.

ERUPTION AND SHEDDING OF THE DECIDUOUS TEETH

	ERUPTION		SHEDDING	
	Lower	Upper	Lower	Upper
	Age	(months)	Age	(years)
Central Incisor	6	7½	6	7½
Lateral Incisor	7	9	7	8
Cuspid	16	18	9½	11½
First Molar	12	14	10	10½
Second Molar	20	24	11	10½
Incisors	Range ± 2 mos.		Range ± 6 mos.	
Molars	Range ± 4 mos.			

Usually the teeth erupt and are shed earlier in slender children than in children of the stocky type.

OCCLUSION OF THE TEETH

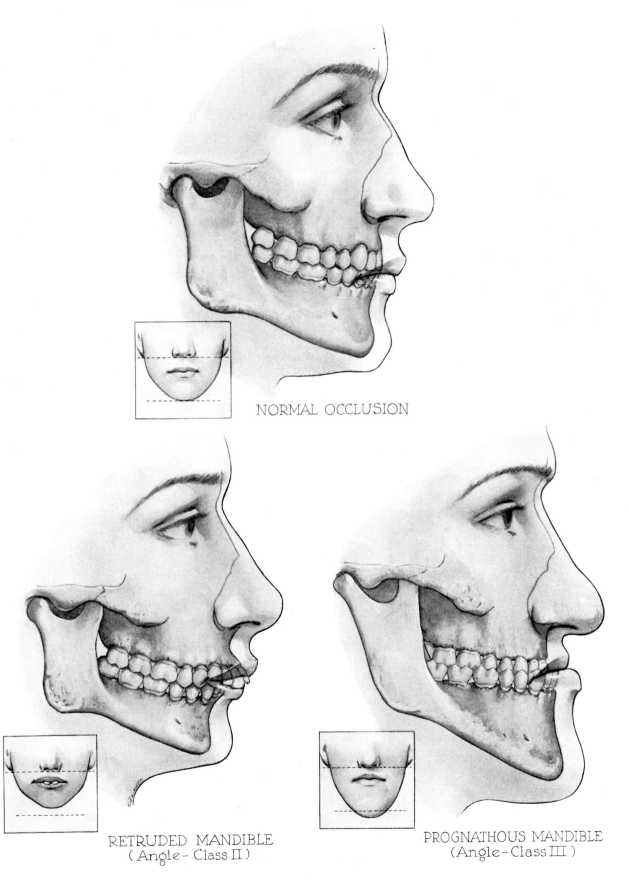

NORMAL OCCLUSION

RETRUDED MANDIBLE
(Angle - Class II)

PROGNATHOUS MANDIBLE
(Angle - Class III)

PLATE 5.

LIFE CYCLE OF THE TOOTH

EACH tooth undergoes the following successive periods of development during its life cycle:

I. GROWTH:

   (A) **Initiation:** Beginning formation of the tooth bud from the oral epithelium.

   (B) **Proliferation:** Multiplication of cells and elaboration of the enamel organ.

   (C) **Histodifferentiation:** Specialization of cells. The cells of the inner epithelium of the enamel organ become ameloblasts; the peripheral cells of the dentin organ (pulp) become odontoblasts.

   (D) **Morphodifferentiation:** Arrangement of formative cells along the future dentino-enamel (and dentino-cemental) junction to outline the future crown (and root).

   (E) **Apposition:** Deposition of the enamel and dentin matrix in incremental layers.

II. CALCIFICATION: Hardening of the matrix by deposition of calcium salts.

III. ERUPTION: Migration of the tooth into the oral cavity.

IV. ATTRITION: Wearing of occlusal and interproximal contact surfaces during function.

All developmental aberrations of the teeth may be classified according to the developmental stage affected.

A CLASSIFICATION OF ABERRATIONS IN TOOTH DEVELOPMENT

| CHARACTER OF DISTURBANCE | GROWTH | | | | | CALCIFICATION | ERUPTION | ATTRITION |
| | INITIATION → PROLIFERATION | HISTODIFFERENTIATION → | MORPHODIFFERENTIATION → | APPOSITION | | | | |
	ABNORMAL NUMBER	ATYPICAL STRUCTURE	ATYPICAL FORMS & SIZES	ABNORMAL AMOUNT		ABNORMAL HARDNESS	ABNORMAL ERUPTION	ABNORMAL WEARING
DEFICIENT DEVELOPMENT	Anodontia- partial or complete Congenital absence of lateral incisors, third molars, bicuspids, etc.	Amelogenesis Imperfecta (Ameloblasts) Dentinogenesis Imperfecta (Odontoblasts) Vitamin A Deficiency (Odontogenic Epithelium)	Peg teeth Hutchinson's incisor Mulberry molars Microdontia	Hypoplasias- systemic or local Chronologic enamel hypoplasia Localized enamel pits Dentin hypoplasia (Pulpal inclusions)		Hypocalcification Mottled (chalky) enamel Malacotic enamel Interglobular dentin	Delayed Eruption of teeth single or multiple Submerged denture Submerged teeth (ankylosis) Impacted teeth Malposed teeth	Deficient Wear Restricted lateral excursion
EXCESSIVE DEVELOPMENT	Epithelial Rests → Odontogenic Epithelium → Odontomes Cysts Adamantinomas Odontocoeles		Extra cusps and roots Dens in Dente Macrodontia Supernumerary Teeth	Enamel nodules Simple, compound and complex odontomes		Sclerotic Dentin resulting from age, injury or caries	Malocclusions Excessive mesial and occlusal drift of teeth Supraocclusion of teeth	Excessive Wear Night grinding (Bruxism)

Reference: SCHOUR, ISAAC, and MASSLER, MAURY: Studies in Tooth Development: The Growth of the Human Teeth. Part I. *J.A.D.A.,* 27:1778-1793, November 1940: II. Ibid., 27: 1918-1931, December 1940.

LIFE CYCLE OF THE TOOTH

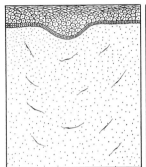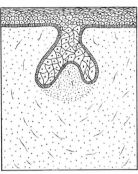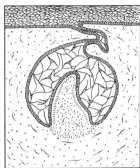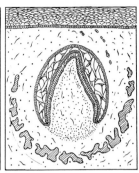

GROWTH

Initiation   Proliferation   Histodifferentiation Morphodifferentiation

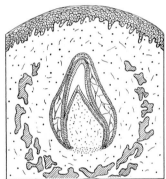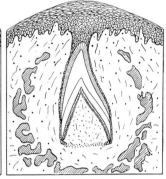

Apposition   CALCIFICATION

Intraosseous eruption

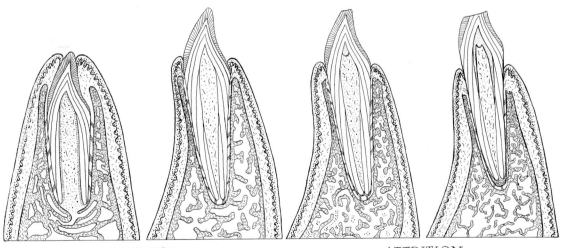

ERUPTION   ATTRITION

(Clinical)   (and continuous eruption)

PLATE 6.

PHYSIOLOGIC SPACING OF THE ANTERIOR TEETH

SPACES between the teeth occur normally at different periods in the development of the dentitions. Such physiologic spacings have been mistaken for abnormalities.

Spacing Associated with Growth of the Jaws

The deciduous denture is in harmony with the size of the jaws of the child from 2 to 5 years of age. As the jaws grow, the anterior teeth of the closed deciduous arch may become spaced in order to rest evenly on its larger base. The jaws grow, but the teeth do not. The deciduous teeth, therefore, are replaced by the larger sized permanent teeth to fit the larger adult jaw.

Spacing of Newly Erupted Anterior Teeth

The crowns of the anterior teeth, both upper and lower, are crowded and are staggered in position while developing within the growing but relatively small jaws. These teeth, when they first erupt into the oral cavity, are still staggered in position and are often incorrect in inclination and even partially rotated.

In addition, the upper central incisors are frequently spaced, resulting in a central diastema. This state is, however, a temporary one and is self-correcting. As they erupt, the permanent upper lateral incisors and cuspids guide the central incisors into better alinement and interproximal contact. Complete closure of the central diastema may not occur until the eruption of the cuspid. The final molding of the arch and the alinement of the teeth are accomplished by the action of the tongue and labial musculature. This process can be readily traced in successive roentgenograms of the same child taken over a period of time. (See bottom of plate.)

The sequence of events is similar when the deciduous anterior teeth, particularly the upper central incisors, first erupt into the oral cavity at from six to nine months of age.

Reference: BROADBENT, B. HOLLY: Ontogenetic Development of Occlusion. Philadelphia: University of Pennsylvania Press, 1941.

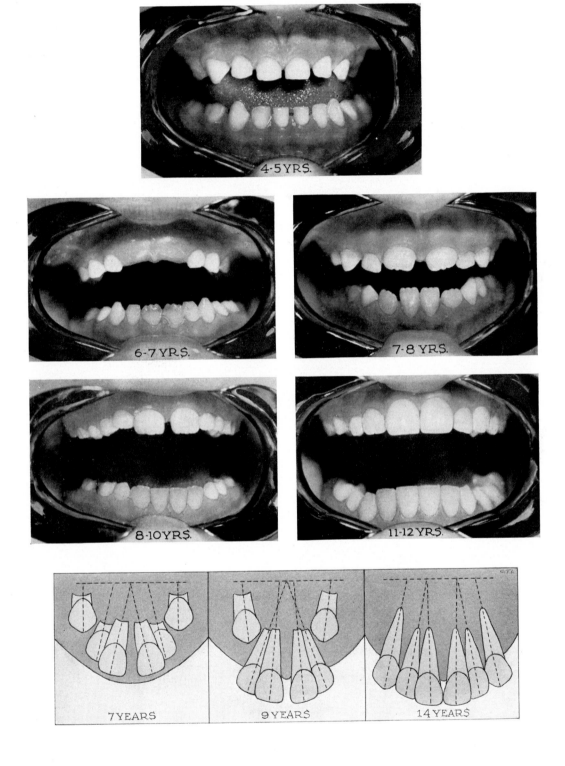

PLATE 7.

DENTAL CARIES

Definition. Dental caries is a progressive lesion of the calcified dental tissues (enamel, dentin or cementum) characterized by loss of tooth structure resulting from a solution of the inorganic and digestion of the organic tooth substances. The exciting cause appears to be a mixed bacterial infection beginning at the surface and progressing toward the pulp.

Sites of Predilection. Areas where bacterial action can proceed undisturbed are quickly attacked by caries (pits and fissures, interproximal areas, bacterial plaques and non-cleansable areas caused by malpositioning of teeth).

Contributory Factors. Neglect and lack of oral hygiene contribute to the progress of caries. So does a diet high in carbohydrates and poor in detergent action.

Age Incidence. No age is free from the disease, but caries activity is highest between 5 and 8, and 12 and 18 years of age. The incidence of new caries lesions decreases after 40 years of age. In later life cemental caries occurs (senile caries).

Prognosis and Treatment. Since dental caries is a disease of a tissue which cannot regenerate or repair itself, the lesion is progressive and the disease is cumulative. It is sometimes self-limiting (arrested caries), but never self-reparative. Repair can be accomplished only by dental restorations. There is therefore no substitute for restorative dentistry.

Control of dental decay requires :

    (1) Early and regular dental examinations and necessary corrections.
    (2) A diet balanced in nutrition and detergent in action.
    (3) Oral hygiene.

ORDINARY (SIMPLE) CARIES

Simple caries occurs in almost all individuals and begins in occlusal grooves and at interproximal contact areas of the posterior teeth.

TEEN-AGE CARIES

A sudden exacerbation of new carious lesions at adolescence, characterized by a rapidly burrowing type of decay. It follows the adolescent spurt in growth and is more marked in the slender type of child.

NEGLECTED CARIES

The carious areas increase in number and extent because of lack of oral hygiene (filth caries) and lack of control by dental treatment.

RAMPANT CARIES

Rampant caries is a very rapid and extensive spread of caries on almost all exposed tooth surfaces, affecting even the lower anterior teeth. Contributory factors are many.

Reference: MASSLER, MAURY, and SCHOUR, ISAAC: The Mouth and Its Diseases.

DENTAL CARIES

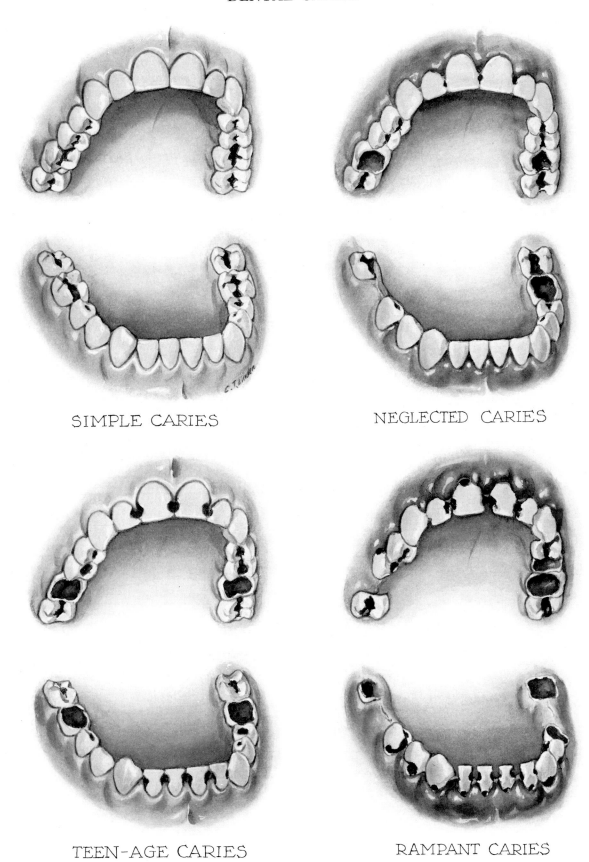

SIMPLE CARIES

NEGLECTED CARIES

TEEN-AGE CARIES

RAMPANT CARIES

PLATE 8.

TEN STAGES IN THE PROGRESS OF DENTAL CARIES

(CLINICAL AND HISTOLOGIC)

STAGE	CLINICAL APPEARANCE	SUBJECTIVE SYMPTOMS	
ENAMEL CARIES			
1. Bacterial colony in groove or on surface of tooth	Debris or bacterial plaque on tooth surface	None	
2. Decalcification of enamel by products of acidogenic organisms	Chalky white opacity of enamel (precarious lesion)	None	
3. Cavitation of enamel	Small cavity in enamel, often detectable only by x-rays.	None	
DENTIN CARIES			
4. Beginning dentin invasion: (a) Decalcification (b) Proteolysis of organic matrix	Small cavity in dentin Cavity beginning to enlarge and become discolored	Sharp lancinating pain, aggravated by thermal shock or ingested sugars or acids	1st warning
5. Continued dentin invasion	Cavity enlarged. Enamel undermined and falls in	Pain (dentinal). "Jumping toothache"	2nd warning
6. Invasion deep into the dentin and approaching the pulp	Large cavity with discoloration	Pain diminishes as dentinal fibers are destroyed	
PULPAL INFECTION			
7. Pulpitis	Deep cavity. Usually filled with necrotic debris	Pain (pulpal)	**Last warning** Tooth can still be saved by pulpectomy and root canal therapy
8. Death of pulp	Tooth becomes discolored	No pain	
PERIAPICAL INFECTION			
9. Localized periapical granuloma, cyst or abscess	Crown of tooth broken down to the gingival line; pulp necrotic	Pain in acute stage; no pain in chronic stage Pain (periapical)	
10. Spreading periapical infection		Tender to pressure	

Reference: NOYES, F. B.; SCHOUR, ISAAC and NOYES, H. J.: A Text-Book of Dental Histology and Embryology. Philadelphia: Lea & Febiger, 1938.

THE PROGRESS OF DENTAL CARIES

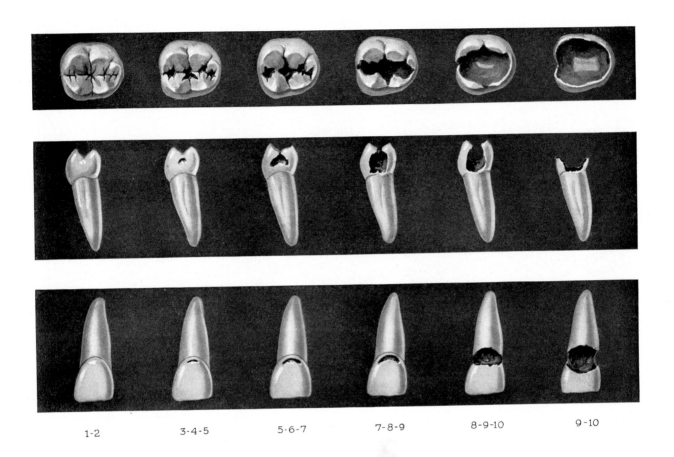

1-2   3-4-5   5-6-7   7-8-9   8-9-10   9-10

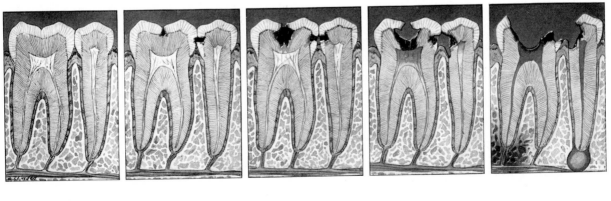

1-2   3-4   5-6   7-8   9-10

PLATE 9.

EFFECTS OF THE LOSS OF A TOOTH

THE dental arch is not a static structure, but rather one that is in a state of dynamic balance among the various forces acting upon it. The removal of a single element in the arch upsets this equilibrium and may result in the breakdown of the entire dental apparatus. The resulting malocclusion leads to improper mastication of the food. Cleansing with the toothbrush is difficult and the normal cleansing action of the food does not occur. The irregularities in the alinement and occlusion of the teeth, therefore, are important predisposing factors in the progress of dental caries and periodontal disease.

The first permanent molar is the keystone of the dental arch. The extraction of a lower first molar without immediate replacement, especially after eruption of the second permanent molar, may result in shifting of the teeth, malocclusion, periodontal injury and caries. These effects tend to develop in the following sequence:

1. Mesial and lingual tilting of the lower second permanent molar into the space left by the lower first permanent molar.
2. Separation of the lower second and third molars followed by food impaction and periodontal injury. The periodontal injury is aggravated by the traumatic occlusion on the distal half of these teeth.
3. Extrusion of upper first permanent molar into the lower molar space, followed eventually by denuding of its palatal root.
4. Increased tilting of upper as well as lower molars as a result of occlusal forces which are no longer transmitted along the long axis of these teeth.
5. Tendency of upper molars to shift buccally as the lower molars tilt lingually.
6. Closing of bite causing shifting of bicuspids and anterior teeth.
7. Tilting of lower second bicuspids into space of lower first molar.
8. Separation between lower bicuspids, leading to food impaction and formation of periodontal pockets.
9. Lingual tilting of lower anterior teeth so that they occlude on the palatal gingivae of the upper anterior teeth with further closing and locking of the bite.

PREMATURE LOSS OF DECIDUOUS TEETH

The deciduous teeth are too often neglected by parents on the premise that they are "temporary" teeth and will soon be lost. The deciduous teeth not only serve in the mastication of food, but also act as space maintainers for their permanent successors. The effects of early loss of a deciduous cuspid or molar tooth may be disastrous, since malocclusion of the entire permanent arch may result. The loss of deciduous incisors rarely has serious consequences.

The results of premature loss of a lower second deciduous molar are, for the most part, similar to those of the loss of a first permanent molar:

1. The lower first permanent molar tilts toward the space left by the lost deciduous molar.
2. The upper deciduous second molar drops down out of line and may become decayed and abscessed.
3. The lower second bicuspid is prevented from erupting properly because its space has become narrowed. It is often forced to erupt buccally or lingually to the rest of the arch.
4. The lower first deciduous molar drifts and tilts into the space left by the lost tooth and the continuity of the entire arch is further destroyed. Caries and periodontal disturbances follow.

Reference: LEONARD, H. J.: Relation of Basic Science to Clinical Dentistry. VIII. Pathology and Oral Anatomy to Periodontology and Prosthodontia. *J. D. Ed.*, 5:40-51, October 1940.

EFFECTS OF THE LOSS OF A TOOTH

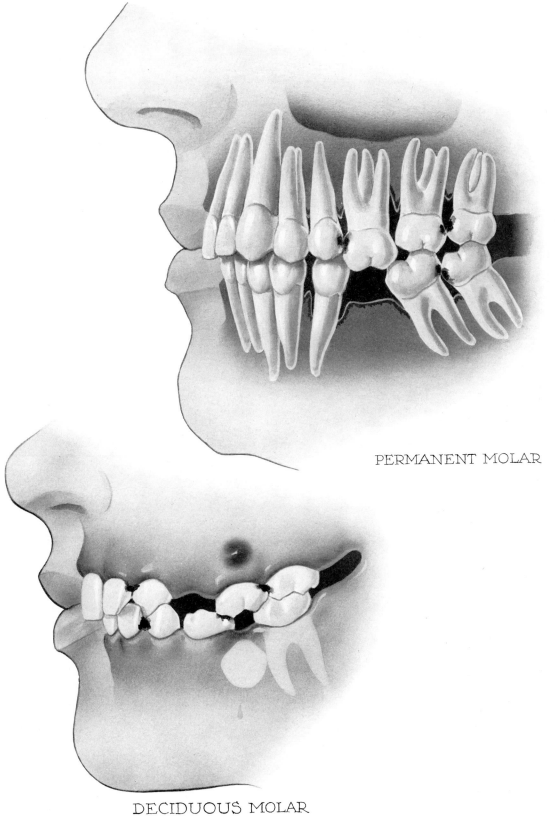

PERMANENT MOLAR

DECIDUOUS MOLAR

PLATE 10.

DENTAL EROSION

Definition. Erosion is a progressive smooth wearing of the tooth structure generally at the gingivolabial or buccal level. This lesion, which may be wedge- or cup-shaped, is characterized by a smooth, hard, highly polished surface, increased sensitivity and no evidence of bacterial action.

Incidence. It begins in the young adult and rises during middle age.

Sites of Predilection. Erosion generally begins in the cuspid-bicuspid region and spreads anteriorly and posteriorly. It commonly begins in the cementum at the cemento-enamel junction.

Etiology. The exact etiologic factors are unknown. The following conditions have been held responsible:
1. Chemical erosion by acid secretions from the labial or buccal mucosal glands. Generally found in nervous, sensitive individuals who are chronic worriers.
2. Mechanical wear resulting from incorrect toothbrushing (cross-brushing) with an abrasive dentifrice. Increased gingival festooning is present.
3. Combinations of 1 and 2. Dental erosion usually proceeds at a more rapid rate than can be explained by incorrect toothbrushing alone and follows a pattern which differs from that produced by toothbrushing.

Progress. The lesion may progress at a very rapid rate. It rarely exposes the pulp because usually the formation of secondary dentin is more rapid and prevents this occurrence. (See insets.) The lesion is not self-reparative, but occasionally is arrested spontaneously and becomes insensitive and discolored.

Configuration Types. The lesion may be:
(1) wedge-shaped or notched,
(2) dish-shaped or saucered or
(3) figured.

Treatment. No effective treatment is known. Metallic fillings may not stop the progress of the erosion, but will change its direction and check deepening, and will protect the tooth against fracture.

Reference: BLACK, G. V.: Operative Dentistry. Vol. 1, Ed. 7, Chicago: Medico-Dental Publishing Co., 1936.

DENTAL EROSION

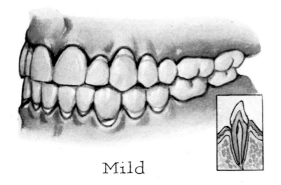

Mild

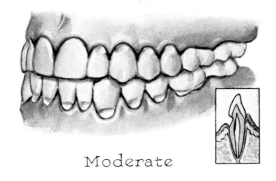

Moderate

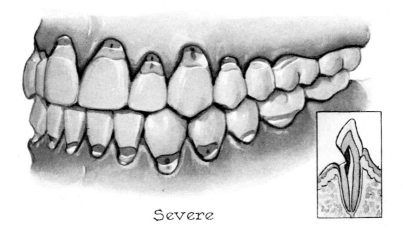

Severe

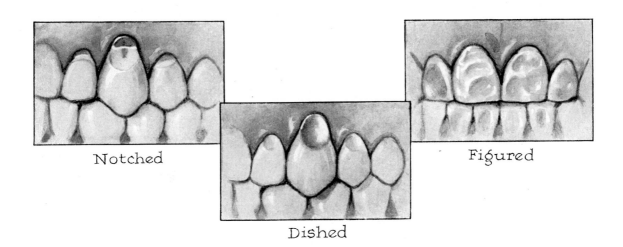

Notched

Dished

Figured

PLATE II.

DENTAL FLUOROSIS

(Mottled Enamel)

DENTAL fluorosis is a developmental disturbance resulting in a poor calcification of the enamel (and dentin). It is caused by the ingestion of excessive amounts of fluorides (more than one part per million of water) during the period of calcification of the developing teeth. Change or chemical treatment of the water supply containing the fluorides is the best preventive.

Mottled enamel is opaque and, in severe cases, it is chalky and crumbles easily, in contrast to normal enamel, which is hard, glossy and translucent.

The fluorides are usually derived from the drinking water obtained from artesian wells in endemic areas. The mottling of the enamel varies in extent and severity, according to the amount of fluorides ingested.

Mild. The enamel shows white opaque areas which involve up to 50 per cent of the tooth surface.

Moderate. The entire enamel surface is affected and brown staining occurs secondarily (from oral pigments) in varying degrees.

Severe. All enamel surfaces show mottling and discrete or confluent hypoplastic pitting is present.

Reference: Dean, H. T.: Investigation of Physiological Effects by Epidemiological Method. Fluorine and Dental Health. Publication of the American Association for the Advancement of Science, No. 19, 1942.

DENTAL FLUOROSIS

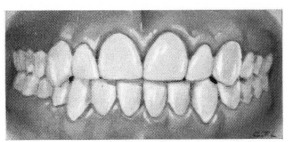

NORMAL

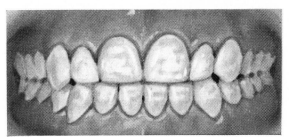

MILD

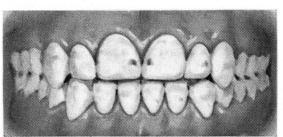

MODERATE

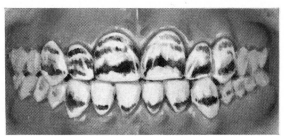

MODERATE

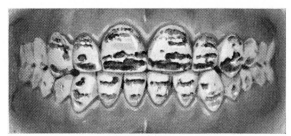

SEVERE

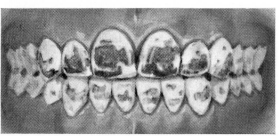

SEVERE

PLATE 12.

CHRONOLOGY OF TOOTH DEVELOPMENT

THE teeth are shown on a chronologic grid to assist in the clinical analysis of the chronology of developmental defects of the teeth, particularly hypoplasia.

The levels of the developmental rings and periods are indicated on the right. (For details, see Plate 14.)

DECIDUOUS DENTITION

	Hard Tissue Formation Begins	Amount of Enamel Formed at Birth	Crown Completed
MAXILLARY	(Months in Utero)		(Months)
Central incisor	4	5/6	1½
Lateral incisor	4½	2/3	2½
Cuspid	5	1/3	9
First molar	5	Cusps united	6
Second molar	6	Cusp tips still isolated	11
MANDIBULAR			
Central incisor	4½	3/5	2½
Lateral incisor	4½	3/5	3
Cuspid	5	1/3	9
First molar	5	Cusps united	5½
Second molar	6	Cusp tips still isolated	10

PERMANENT DENTITION

	Hard Tissue Formation Begins	Crown Completed	Root Completed
MAXILLARY		(Years)	(Years)
First molar*	At birth	2½- 3	9-10
Central incisor	3- 4 mos.	4 - 5	10
Lateral incisor	10-12 mos.	4 - 5	11
Cuspid	4- 5 mos.	6 - 7	13-15
First bicuspid	1½-1¾ yrs.	5 - 6	12-13
Second bicuspid	2 -2¼ yrs.	6 - 7	12-14
Second molar	2½-3 yrs.	7 - 8	14-16
Third molar	7 -9 yrs.	12 -16	18-25
MANDIBULAR			
First molar	At birth	2½- 3	9-10
Central incisor	3-4 mos.	4 - 5	9
Lateral incisor	3-4 mos.	4 - 5	10
Cuspid	4-5 mos.	6 - 7	12-14
First bicuspid	1¾- 2 yrs.	5 - 6	12-13
Second bicuspid	2¼- 2½ yrs.	6 - 7	13-14
Second molar	2½- 3 yrs.	7 - 8	14-15
Third molar	8 -10 yrs.	12 -16	18-25

*The first permanent molar is placed first since chronologically it is the first permanent tooth and developmentally the last deciduous tooth.

Reference: LOGAN, W. H. G. and KRONFELD, RUDOLF: Development of Human Jaws and Surrounding Structures from Birth to Age of 15 Years. *J.A.D.A.,* 20:379-427, March 1933.

CHRONOLOGY OF TOOTH DEVELOPMENT

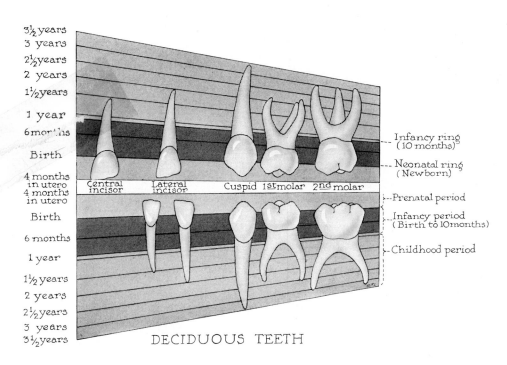

3½ years
3 years
2½ years
2 years
1½ years
1 year
6 months
Birth
4 months in utero
4 months in utero
Birth
6 months
1 year
1½ years
2 years
2½ years
3 years
3½ years

Central incisor   Lateral incisor   Cuspid 1st molar 2nd molar

Infancy ring (10 months)
Neonatal ring (Newborn)
Prenatal period
Infancy period (Birth to 10 months)
Childhood period

DECIDUOUS TEETH

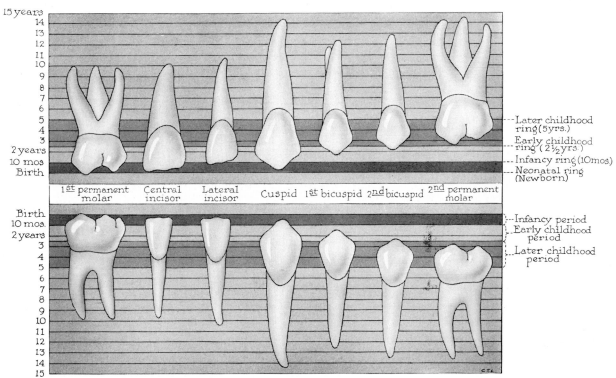

15 years
14
13
12
11
10
9
8
7
6
5
4
3
2 years
10 mos.
Birth

1st permanent molar   Central incisor   Lateral incisor   Cuspid 1st bicuspid 2nd bicuspid 2nd permanent molar

Later childhood ring (5 yrs.)
Early childhood ring (2½ yrs.)
Infancy ring (10 mos.)
Neonatal ring (Newborn)

Birth
10 mos.
2 years
3
4
5
6
7
8
9
10
11
12
13
14
15

Infancy period
Early childhood period
Later childhood period

PERMANENT TEETH

PLATE 13.

GROWTH AND CALCIFICATION PATTERNS OF ENAMEL AND DENTIN

A DIAGRAMMATIC representation of the calcification pattern is superposed on the incremental growth pattern and its chronology. The teeth are shown in labiolingual section.

DEVELOPMENTAL PATTERN OF THE CHILD AND ITS REFLECTION IN THE TEETH

Developmental Periods and Tooth Rings	Age Period	Physiologic and Developmental Characteristics	Quality of Calcification and Histologic Characteristics of the Enamel and Dentin
Prenatal Period	In utero	Well-protected parasitic existence	Homogeneous calcification; disturbed calcification and enamel hypoplasias rare
Neonatal Ring	Birth to 2 weeks	Neonatal adjustments; birth trauma; arrest in growth	Dark, distinct arrest line in enamel and dentin
Infancy Period	2 weeks to about 10 months	Period of postnatal adjustment; marked susceptibility to infection; alimentary and metabolic disturbances	Period of poorest calcification and greatest susceptibility to chronic hypoplastic defects
Infancy Ring	About 10 months	Time of greatest susceptibility to diseases of infancy; a "critical" period; temporary depression in growth curve	Sharp arrest line which demarcates infancy from early childhood and marks a period of acute susceptibility to hypoplastic defects of enamel as well as abrupt termination of chronic hypoplastic defects of infancy
Early Childhood Period	About 10 months to 2½ years	More independent existence; improved alimentation and antibody mechanism	Cessation of hypoplasia abrupt and complete; calcification better than during infancy, but not so good as during prenatal period; hypoplasia relatively rare
Early Childhood Ring	About 2½ years	?	Sharp arrest line which separates early and later childhood periods and marks a period of acute susceptibility to enamel hypoplasia
Later Childhood Period	About 2½ to 5 years	Most of the exanthematous and other diseases of childhood occur during this period	Calcification generally poor, but better than during infancy period; chronic hypoplasia somewhat more common
Later Childhood Ring	About 5 years	?	A sharp arrest line which demarcates the later childhood from the grade-school period and marks a period of acute susceptibility to enamel hypoplasia
Grade-School Age	About 5 to 10 years	?	Calcification generally good, but variable; hypoplasia rare

The levels of teeth affected are given in Plates 13 and 15. The registration period in teeth is virtually ended after the tenth year.

Because of the extreme sensitivity of the enamel-forming cells to metabolic disturbances, severe disturbances in calcification are manifested also in deficient enamel formation (enamel hypoplasia), which can be recognized grossly. (Plate 15.)

Reference: MASSLER, MAURY; SCHOUR, ISAAC, and PONCHER, H. G.: Developmental Pattern of the Child as Reflected in the Calcification Pattern of the Teeth. *Am. J. Dis. Child.*, 62:33-67, July 1941.

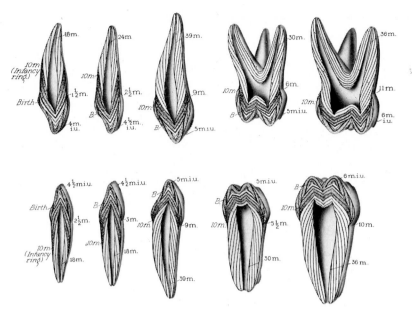

DECIDUOUS TEETH

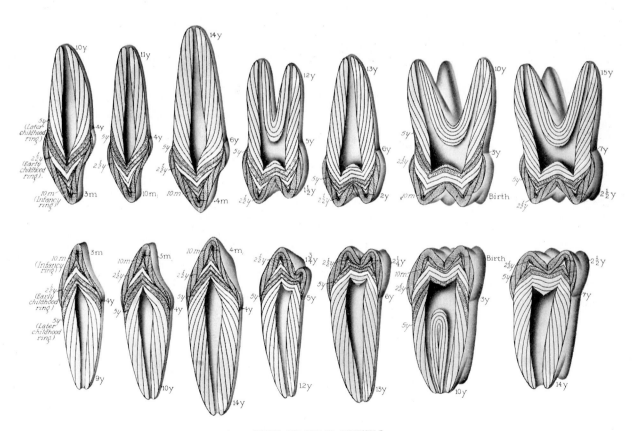

PERMANENT TEETH

PLATE 14.

ENAMEL HYPOPLASIA

ENAMEL hypoplasia is a deficient formation of the enamel matrix due to injury to the ameloblasts (enamel-forming cells) during enamel formation. It is seen clinically as a pitting or grooving of the enamel at homologous chronologic levels of all the teeth forming at that time. The effect may be acute (short duration) or chronic (longer duration).

From 5 to 10 per cent of the total population are affected. The incidence is higher in rural than in urban communities.

The hypoplastic defects are analogous to the lines of arrested growth seen at the epiphyseal ends of the growing long bones. The scarring in the enamel is: (a) permanent, (b) easily recognized clinically and (c) easily assessed chronologically. (Plate 13.)

TYPE OF HYPOPLASIA	INCIDENCE* AND TEETH AFFECTED†						ETIOLOGY
Neonatal Hypoplasia	10%						Birth trauma resulting in disturbances of neonatal adjustment
	I	II	III	IV	V	6	
	a	b	c	d	e	6	
Acute Hypoplasia of the Infancy Ring (10 months)	30%						Some acute metabolic upset, usually subclinical and of unknown origin
	I		3			6	
	I	2	3			6	
Chronic Hypoplasia of the Infancy Period (birth to 10 months)	40%						(a) Continuation of unsatisfactory neonatal adjustment
	I		3				(b) Diarrhea and vomiting Feeding difficulties
	I	II	III	IV	V	6	(c) Infantile tetany, rickets, parathyroprivic tetany, etc.
	a	b	c	d	e	6	(d) Rarely exanthemas
	I	2	3				(e) Congenital syphilis

The hypoplasia usually stops suddenly at 10 months of age; the clinical symptoms may or may not stop suddenly

TYPE OF HYPOPLASIA	INCIDENCE* AND TEETH AFFECTED†	ETIOLOGY
Acute Hypoplasia of the Early and Later Childhood Rings (2½ and 4½ years)	10% — All permanent teeth	Acute disturbances of childhood (exanthemas)
Chronic Hypoplasia of the Childhood Period (2½ - 4½ years)	5% — All permanent teeth	Chronic diseases of childhood
Recurrent Hypoplasia	Rare — All permanent teeth	Unknown

*Percentage of total number of cases of enamel hypoplasia observed.
†For teeth and levels affected, see Plates 13 and 14.

Reference: SARNAT, B. G., and SCHOUR, ISAAC: Enamel Hypoplasia (Chronologic Enamel Aplasia) in Relation to Systemic Disease: Chronologic, Morphologic and Etiologic Classification. Part I *J.A.D.A.*, **28**:1989-2000, December 1941; Part II Ibid., **29**:67-75, January 1942.

ENAMEL HYPOPLASIA

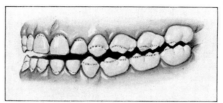

Neonatal hypoplasia

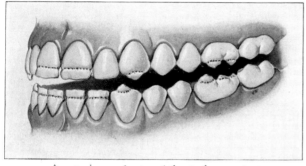

Acute hypoplasia of the infancy ring
(10 mos.)

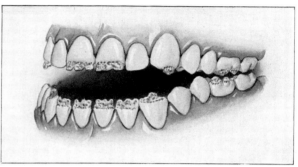

Chronic hypoplasia of the infancy period
(Birth to 10 mos.)

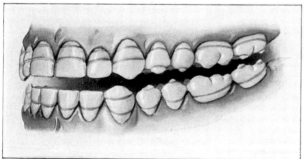

Acute hypoplasia of the early and later childhood rings
(2½ and 4½ years)

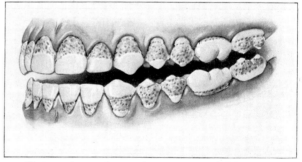

Chronic hypoplasia of the childhood period
(2½ to 4½ years)

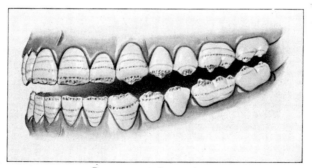

Recurrent hypoplasia

PLATE 15.

THE TEETH IN CONGENITAL SYPHILIS

CONGENITAL syphilis, an infectious disease contracted sometimes during birth, is exacerbated during the neonatal and early infancy periods. The disease can affect only the teeth developing at that time and only the particular stage of current development. Therefore, the permanent incisors, cuspids and first molars, which are at the stage of *morphodifferentiation* at the time of the exacerbation, show a disturbance in *tooth form;* the deciduous teeth, which are active in the *formation of enamel* and dentin show *hypoplastic defects,* but no effects upon tooth form; whereas the bicuspids and permanent second and third molars, which are still in the bud stage, are usually not affected at all. (see also Plate 6.)

In congenital syphilis, the permanent incisors are characteristically abnormal in form, the crown converging instead of diverging incisally (screw-driver shape). The middle developmental lobe may, in addition, particularly in the upper central incisor, actually be missing, a central notch resulting (Hutchinson's incisor). The lower permanent incisors are less frequently affected. The first permanent molars also show a constricted and dwarfed crown, the cusps being relatively crowded.

In addition to the pathognomonic changes in the form of the tooth, the syphilitic condition may (especially when aggravated by other disturbances during infancy) affect the ameloblasts when they begin to form the enamel. This results in a superposition of typical hypoplastic defects upon the original screw-driver-shaped crown.

DIFFERENTIAL DIAGNOSIS

Mammelons. The three mammelons on the incisal edge of newly erupted incisors are remnants of the three developmental lobes or centers in the tooth germ and are a feature of the normal form of these teeth. They soon wear away and the incisal edges become flat. The unworn mammelons may sometimes be mistaken for notched incisors by those unfamiliar with dental anatomy.

Occupational Notches. Notched incisors may result from abrasive action on the teeth such as occurs in upholsterers who hold nails between their incisor teeth during their work. (Plate 18.)

Infancy Hypoplasia. Hypoplastic teeth are sometimes mistaken for syphilitic incisors. When hypoplasia is caused by congenital syphilis, the proximal surfaces converge incisally. If it is caused by other disturbances during infancy, the proximal surfaces do not converge to a screwdriver shape.

Reference: SARNAT, B. G., and SHAW, N. G.: Dental Development in Congenital Syphilis. *Am. J. Dis. Child.,* **64**:771-788, November 1942.

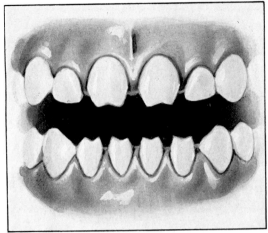

Syphilitic Incisors

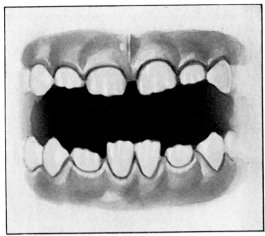

Newly Erupted Incisors
(Showing Mammelons)

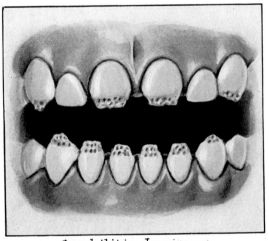

Syphilitic Incisors
with Hypoplasia

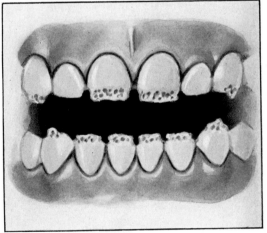

Non-specific Hypoplasia
of Infancy

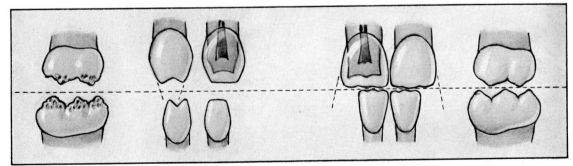

Syphilitic   Normal

PLATE 16.

COMMON LESIONS OF THE BUCCAL MUCOSA

BULLOUS LESIONS (Blister-like Lesions)

Pemphigus. A constant succession of blisters in all stages of development, surrounded by an inflammatory halo and filled with a yellow-brown (bloody) fluid. Blisters break, leaving erosions covered with crusts. There may also be lesions on the skin. There is a nauseating odor from the mouth and skin lesions. The prognosis is very poor.

Erythema Multiforme. Characterized by areas of redness with superposed blisters. Lasts from 2 to 4 weeks and is recurrent in spring and fall. It does not affect health. Skin lesions are also present (dorsal surfaces of the hands and feet and extensor surface of the forearm).

Stomatitis Medicamentosa. Reddish eruptions appearing soon after taking a drug to which one is sensitive. The skin may itch.

WHITISH LESIONS

MEMBRANOUS LESIONS

(Lesions which peel off readily
and leave a raw surface)

Aphthae (Canker Sores). Small, sharply circumscribed ovoid erosions covered with a yellowish white membrane and surrounded by a bright red areola. They are extremely painful and appear suddenly, lasting about ten days. The muco-buccal fold, muco-cutaneous junction of lip and sides of tongue are the sites of predilection.

Mucous Patch (Secondary Syphilis). Infiltrated papules covered with dirty, grayish white membrane. Usually no red areola or pain is present. They follow the appearance of a chancre, appearing suddenly, and are not transitory.

Thrush (Moniliasis). Smooth, white, sharply defined, slightly raised patch which looks like milk curd. It has no inflammatory base and begins as tiny spots which enlarge at the periphery. It occurs more often in infants and debilitated elderly individuals, but may also affect other adults. It is caused by the fungus *Monilia albicans.*

NON-MEMBRANOUS LESIONS

(Solid lesions which do not peel off
and are usually painless)

Leukoplakia (Hyperkeratosis). Distinctly elevated leathery patches irregular in outline and bluish white or grayish white in color. It develops slowly and remains for a long time.

Lichen Planus. A fine lacework of pearly-white lines with nodes at the intersections forms a mosaic inlay pattern. It is not elevated and is generally associated with skin lesions.

Cheek-Biting. The cheek lining is ragged and torn. There is a history of trauma.

Reference: EPSTEIN, C. M., and SENEAR, F. E.: Stomatitis, in Tice's Practice of Medicine. Hagerstown, Md.: W. F. Prior Co., 1940.

COMMON LESIONS OF THE BUCCAL MUCOSA

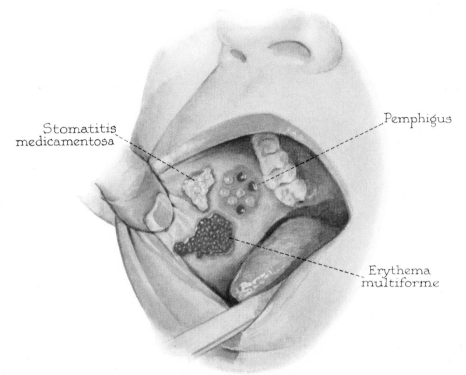

Stomatitis
medicamentosa

Pemphigus

Erythema
multiforme

BULLOUS LESIONS

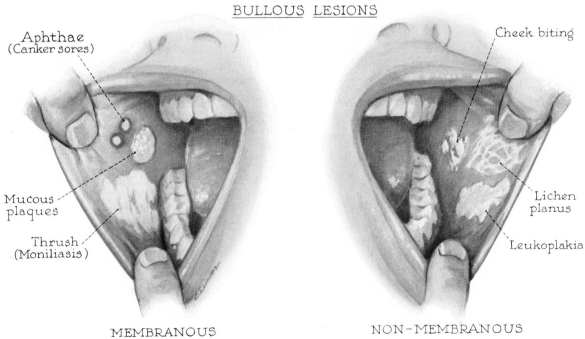

Aphthae
(Canker sores)

Cheek biting

Mucous
plaques

Lichen
planus

Thrush
(Moniliasis)

Leukoplakia

MEMBRANOUS

NON-MEMBRANOUS

WHITISH LESIONS

PLATE 17.

COMMON LESIONS OF THE LIPS

FISSURES

Angular Fissures. Maceration and scaling leading to fissuring at the angles of the mouth. It may be caused by yeast infection (perlèche), riboflavin deficiency (cheilosis) or a closed bite in elderly edentulous persons (mechanical fissures).

Cheilitis. Dryness followed by scaling and cracking of the vermilion border of the lips and accompanied by a characteristic burning sensation.

EROSIONS AND ULCERS

Syphilitic Lesions. The chancre of primary syphilis is a smooth, round, painless ulcer exuding sero-pus teeming with spirochetes. The secondary lesions may be simple spots, gray craters (split papules) at the inside corners of the mouth or mucous patches (see Plate 17). The tertiary lesions (gummas) may be localized (hard, painless nodules which ulcerate and become necrotic) or diffuse (large ulcerations, necrosis of bone, etc). Digital infection is an occupational hazard for which the dentist must be ever watchful.

Aphthous Ulcer (Canker Sore). (See Plate 17.)

SWELLINGS

Tumors. Solid, cellular growths. The most common benign types are the papilloma and the verruca (wart).

The early diagnosis of malignant tumors is one of the major responsibilities of the dentist to his patient and his medical colleagues. The lower lip is a frequent site of carcinoma.

Fordyce's disease may be included here although it is neither a disease nor a tumor but a patch of pinhead-sized yellowish points on the superficial mucosa formed by aberrant sebaceous glands. It is very common and no treatment is indicated.

Bullous Lesions. Circumscribed swellings filled with fluid. The most common types found on the lips are herpes simplex (fever blisters), allergic eruptions and the mucous retention cyst.

Edema. A sudden diffuse swelling of the lip (usually the upper) which returns to normal in a short time. It may be caused by trauma, insect bites or by neurogenic conditions (angioneurotic edema). Occasionally, the swelling may become permanent and the lip solid and rubbery (macrochelia).

Reference: PRINZ, HERMANN, and GREENBAUM, S. S.: Diseases of the Mouth and Their Treatment. Ed. 2. Philadelphia: Lea and Febiger, 1939.

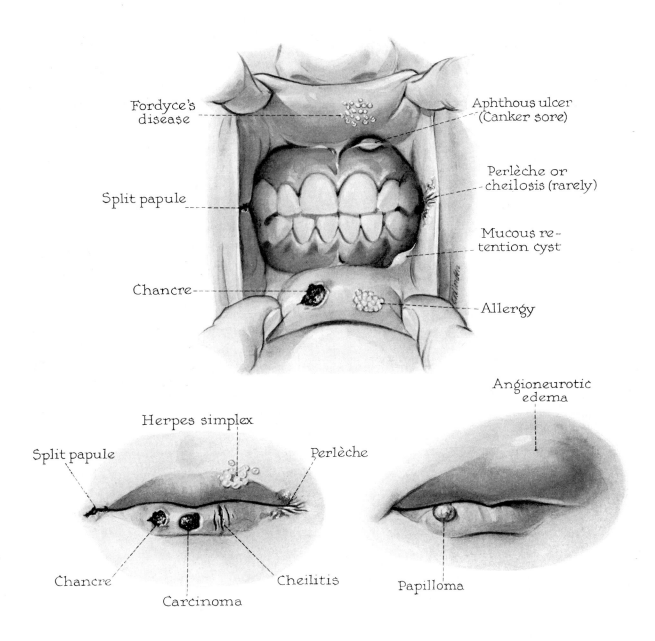

Fordyce's disease

Split papule

Chancre

Aphthous ulcer (Canker sore)

Perlèche or cheilosis (rarely)

Mucous retention cyst

Allergy

Angioneurotic edema

Split papule

Herpes simplex

Perlèche

Chancre

Carcinoma

Cheilitis

Papilloma

PLATE 18.

THE PROGRESS OF PERIODONTAL DISEASE

DISTURBANCES of the periodontal tissues (gingivae, periodontal membrane, cementum and alveolar bone) supporting and investing the teeth occur in from 75 to 80% of the adult population. The incidence rises with age. More teeth are lost as a result of periodontal disturbances than from caries.

Periodontal disease may be caused by:
    (1) Local conditions such as calculus, filth and irritation (Simple Gingivitis);
    (2) Systemic conditions that lower tissue resistance (Systemic Gingivitis);
    (3) Combinations of local and systemic conditions (Complex Gingivitis).

FILTH GINGIVITIS (Leading to Periodontitis)

Filth gingivitis is a chronic inflammation of the gingivae caused by irritants (supragingival or subgingival calculus, soft débris or bacteria) at the necks of the teeth. At least fifty per cent of the adult population are affected. If neglected, the chronic gingivitis will lead to (1) resorption of the alveolar crest, (2) gingival recession or pocket formation, (3) mobility of the tooth resulting from the progressive bone destruction and finally (4) loss of the tooth by exfoliation. The only effective treatment is a thorough scaling of all the teeth combined with good oral hygiene.

ALVEOLAR CREST ATROPHY WITH GINGIVAL RECESSION

A slow, progressive resorption of the alveolar crest with mild gingival recession is normal in middle-aged adults. However, local conditions such as poor toothbrushing or abnormal stresses and unknown constitutional factors may result in its premature appearance in the young adult. Pocket formation is rare. It tends to be self-arresting.

DIFFUSE ALVEOLAR ATROPHY (Periodontosis)

Periodontosis is characterized by a progressive, degenerative destruction of the alveolar bone. The condition is probably systemic in nature and tends to affect young adult females more than males. The first clinical sign is usually a migration and spacing of the upper anterior teeth. There is no primary inflammation of the gingivae, no pain, no recession and no pocket formation. The resorption of the alveolar bone begins on the periodontal surface detaching the periodontal fibers and loosening the tooth and may continue until the tooth is exfoliated. The prognosis is questionable but the progress may slow down for no apparent reason.

Reference: GOLDMAN, H. M.: Periodontia. St. Louis: C. V. Mosby Co., 1942.

THE PROGRESS OF PERIODONTAL DISEASE

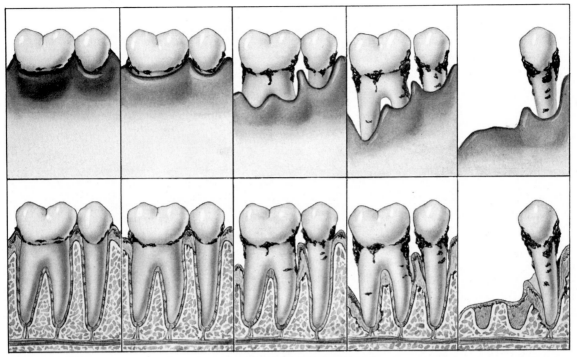

FILTH GINGIVITIS

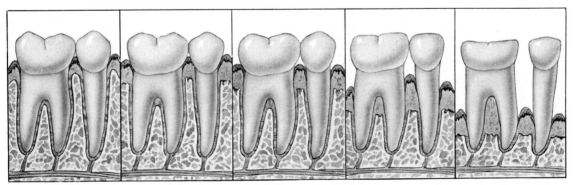

ALVEOLAR CREST ATROPHY

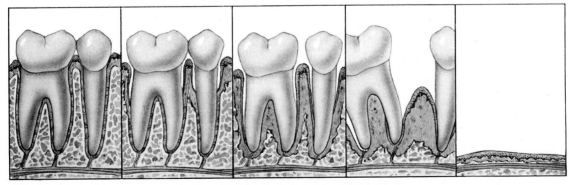

DIFFUSE ALVEOLAR ATROPHY

PLATE 19.

DORSUM OF THE TONGUE

THE tongue is an active and agile mass of voluntary muscle attached posteriorly at the base and free at the anterior apex. The mass of the tongue is composed of intrinsic musculature, so arranged as to permit the tongue to change its shape and size readily and swiftly, and of extrinsic musculature (hyoglossus, genioglossus and styloglossus), which can change the position of this fluid mass swiftly, giving to the whole extreme flexibility. The attachment at only one end makes for increased mobility.

The tongue is covered by a rather thick, highly specialized epithelium which gives it a grayish cast in contrast to the lively red of the rest of the oral mucous membrane.

Functions. The tongue aids in (a) speech, (b) mastication (by crushing and kneading the food against the hard palate and by rolling the bolus of food between the teeth), (c) deglutition (by pressing the food against the hard palate and backward into the oropharynx) and (d) taste. Only in speech is the tongue irreplaceable, since men from whom the tongue has been cut can masticate and swallow food by action of the floor of the mouth and the cheeks.

Circumvallate Papillae. Large round elevated papillae arranged in a V-shaped line (about ten) at the posterior end of the body of the tongue, separating the base from the free portion of the tongue. Each papilla is surrounded by a circular moat both of whose walls contain the taste buds. (See inset.)

Filiform Papillae. Tall, thin, cone-shaped elevations directed backward and covered with numerous fringes composed of hornified epithelium. (See inset.) The latter give the papillae their grayish appearance. They are the most numerous of the lingual papillae and are especially concentrated in a triangular area in front of the circumvallate papillae.

Fungiform Papillae. Squat mushroom-shaped papillae covered with a thin layer of epithelium. They therefore appear as small red mushrooms scattered among the filiform papillae, especially near the lateral margins of the tongue. They readily become engorged under certain conditions, giving to the tongue a raspberry or strawberry appearance. (Plate 22.)

Taste Areas. A substance must be dissolved before it can stimulate the taste buds on the tongue. There are four primary taste sensations; sweet, sour (acid), salty and bitter. The sensation of taste is markedly enhanced by the olfactory sense (sense of smell).

The filiform papillae rarely have taste buds. The fungiform papillae have from eight to ten taste buds in the epithelium of the free surface. These taste buds respond to sweet, sour (acid) or salty materials. Each papillae responds to two of these stimuli, rarely to all three. The circumvallate papillae contain taste buds which respond to bitter stimuli only. The middle third of the dorsum of the tongue is usually taste-free.

Reference: FITZWILLIAMS, D. C. L.: The Tongue and Its Diseases. London: Oxford University Press, 1927.

DORSUM OF THE TONGUE

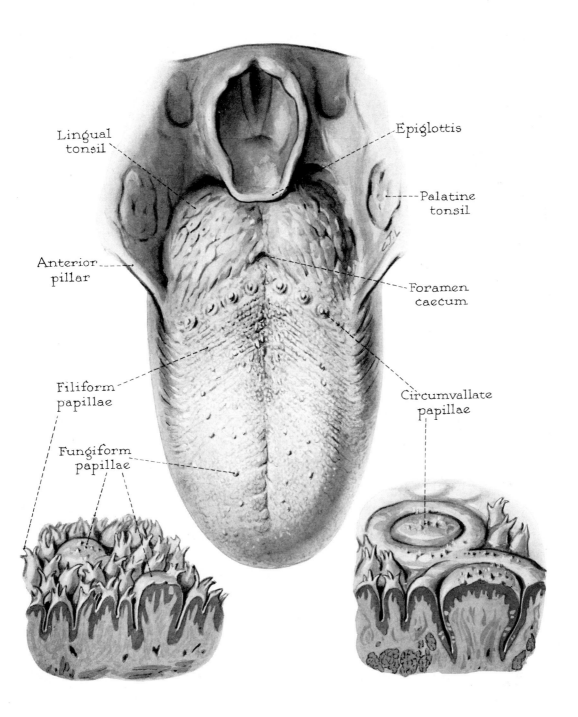

Lingual tonsil

Epiglottis

Palatine tonsil

Anterior pillar

Foramen caecum

Filiform papillae

Circumvallate papillae

Fungiform papillae

PLATE 20.

BENIGN CONDITIONS OF THE TONGUE

THE tongue in certain cases may assume an unusual appearance which is not necessarily pathologic. If the condition is benign, there are no subjective symptoms. The patient is often not even aware of the unusual appearance of his tongue, and it should not be brought to his attention lest a phobia develop. No treatment is indicated or desirable.

Fissured Tongue. A tongue crossed by many deep grooves in a regular or irregular pattern is said to be fissured. The pattern may be foliaceous (leaf-like) or cerebriform. The tongue may be somewhat enlarged and show imprints of the teeth at the sides. Fissured (scrotal) tongue is usually congenital but may be acquired.

Black Hairy Tongue (Lingua Nigra). A condition characterized by an elongation of the filiform papillae into hairlike projections as long as $\frac{1}{2}$ to 1 inch. It is generally concentrated in a triangular area in front of the V-shaped line of circumvallate papillae. The patch may vary from brown to black. The condition is usually chronic and often disappears spontaneously.

Geographic Tongue (Wandering Rash). A tongue characterized by one or more smooth bright-red patches often showing a yellowish or whitish membranous margin upon the dorsum of an otherwise normally roughened tongue. The patches represent areas in which the filiform papillae have become completely desquamated, leaving a smooth, slick surface. The patches may be single or multiple, discrete or confluent (map-like), regular or irregular in outline. They "travel" by extension of desquamation of the papillae at one edge and regeneration of the normal papillae at the other. The patches generally begin at the posterior portion of the tongue in front of the circumvallate papillae, "traveling" anteriorly and laterally until they reach the edge of the tongue and disappear, while a new patch begins in front of the circumvallate papillae. A single cycle may last from two to seven days. The condition is usually chronic.

Reference: SPENCER, W. G., and CADE, S.: Diseases of the Tongue. Ed. 3. Philadelphia: P. Blakiston's Son & Co., 1931.

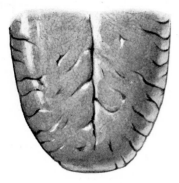

Fissured tongue
Foliaceous type

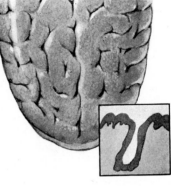

Fissured tongue
Cerebriform type

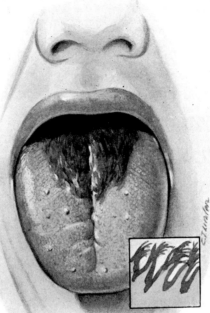

Black hairy tongue

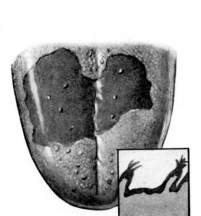

1st stage

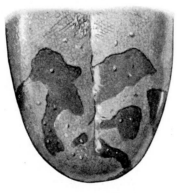

2nd stage
Geographic tongue

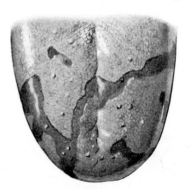

3rd stage

PLATE 21.

THE TONGUE IN SYSTEMIC DISTURBANCES

THE TONGUE reflects changes in the physical state of the body in a vivid and often diagnostic manner. The dental practitioner can obtain much useful information concerning the health of his patient by a careful examination of the tongue.

THE WHITE COATED TONGUE

The Furry Tongue is seen early and often in states of mild dehydrations and low-grade fevers. The fur is actually the hypertrophied filiform papillae. The tongue "tastes" dry.

The Moist Coated Tongue is caused by the accumulation of food débris and bacteria among the hypertrophied filiform papillae. A slight coat is normal in adults in the morning, particularly after an evening of overindulgence and late hours. Unless the tongue is also dry, coating is of little clinical significance.

The Dry Coated Tongue (crusted tongue) is caused by a failure in the secretion of the salivary and lingual glands. Dryness of the tongue is the best clinical index of the state of hydration of the body. It is seen early in all states which tend to cause dehydration (infectious diseases, chronic debilitating diseases, prolonged fevers (not acute), rheumatic fever, gastro-enteritis and after surgery). The color may vary from white to brown.

The White Strawberry Tongue is a transitional stage from the white coated tongue to the raw, red tongue. The appearance is that of an unripe strawberry. The engorged and enlarged fungiform papillae appear prominently above the level of the white desquamating filiform papillae. It is seen early in scarlet fever and other acute febrile states.

THE RAW RED TONGUE (GLOSSITIS)

The Red Raspberry Tongue results when the filiform papillae of the white strawberry tongue or the coated tongue are shed, leaving the engorged fungiform papillae raised above the smooth denuded surface of the tongue. The raspberry tongue is seen often in the later stages of the febrile states.

The Raw Pebbly Tongue (magenta glossitis) results when the papillae become flattened and edematous (mushroom shaped) but not atrophied or shed. The color is a characteristic purplish-red (magenta) instead of pink. Edema of the tongue is common and the indentations of the teeth can easily be seen. The edges of the tongue often become denuded and raw, giving to the tongue a burning, painful sensation. Fissuring is common.

The magenta glossitis is very typical and often diagnostic of ariboflavinosis (riboflavin [vitamin B2] deficiency) when associated with cheilosis and capillary dilatation and proliferation in the eyes. A rapid blanching of the tongue occurs after riboflavin therapy.

A granular glossitis is often found in both chronic gastro-intestinal disease and in chronic alcoholics in whom a riboflavin deficiency often coexists. The purplish-red, pebbly tongue is also seen in thin, nervous women 40 to 50 years of age who complain of glossodynia (burning tongue).

The Smooth Atrophic Tongue (atrophic glossitis) is the result of a complete atrophy of both the filiform and fungiform papillae. The tongue also shrinks in size. The desquamated surface is usually very dry and extremely sensitive to painful stimuli (glazed tongue).

Atrophic glossitis with a fiery-red (scarlet) coloration of the tongue is characteristic of niacin deficiency (pellagrous glossitis) especially when accompanied by ulcerations and Vincent's infections, tenderness and pain. A dramatic recovery in the color and the ulcerations occurs after niacin (nicotinic acid) therapy.

Atrophic glossitis with a pale salmon coloration of the tongue (Hunter's glossitis) is characteristic and often pathognomonic of pernicious anemia. Atrophic glossitis is also seen in sprue, in achlorhydria (raw, red tongue; raw, red gut) and in idiopathic hypochromic anemia of women. Moeller's glossitis is a painful, patchy form of atrophic glossitis whose etiology and treatment are unknown.

The tongue becomes smooth and atrophic in the aged, particularly in those wearing full dentures (bald tongue, slick tongue). Sensitiveness and abnormal taste sensations frequently accompany the senile glossitis.

Reference: JEGHERS, HAROLD: Nutrition: The Appearance of the Tongue as an Index of Nutritional Deficiency. New Eng. Journ. of Med. 227:221-228, Aug. 6, 1942.

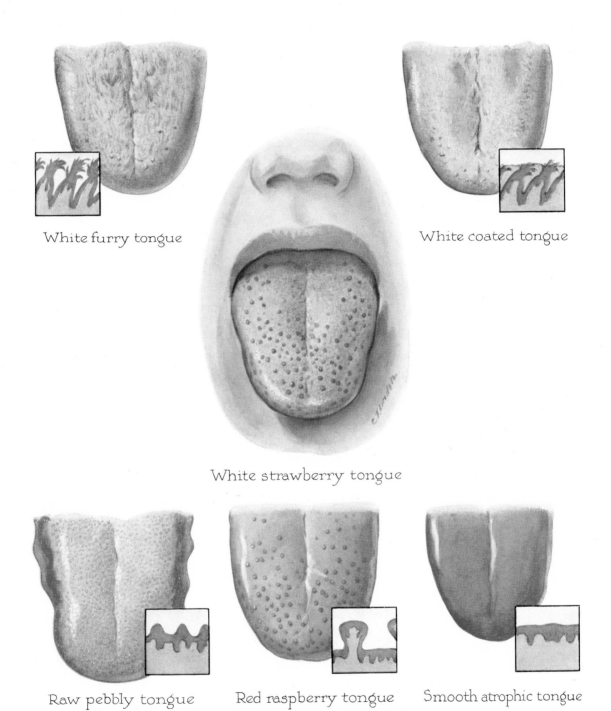

White furry tongue

White coated tongue

White strawberry tongue

Raw pebbly tongue

Red raspberry tongue

Smooth atrophic tongue

PLATE 22.

ORAL DISEASE OF OCCUPATIONAL ORIGIN

ORAL disease of occupational origin rarely occurs in a healthy mouth. In a neglected mouth, even minor systemic ailments will often cause widespread tissue destruction. Oral hygiene is therefore dentistry's contribution to the reduction of occupational disease.

OCCUPATION	ACTIVE AGENT	POSSIBLE ORAL MANIFESTATION
Abrasive powder workers	Dust	Generalized abrasion of teeth
Acid dippers	Fumes	Decalcification of teeth
Arsenic handlers	Arsenic	Necrosis of mandible
Aviators	Atmospheric pressure	Hemorrhage from gingivae, Pulpitis
Bakery workers	Flour, sugar	Calculus, periodontitis, caries
Candy workers	Sugar	Caries
Carpenters.	Nails	Localized abrasion of teeth
Coal tar workers.	Tar	Carcinoma
Cryolite workers	Fluorine	Osteosclerosis
Electrotypers	Lead	Lead line in gingivae
Explosive workers	Benzene	Hemorrhage from gingivae
Garment workers	Chemicals, foreign bodies	Stomatitis, abrasion of teeth
Glass workers	Hydrofluoric acid, increased intraoral pressure	Decalcification, pneumatocele, abrasion
Lead workers	Lead	Lead line in gingivae
Metal workers	Dust (iron, copper, chromium)	Staining of enamel
Mercury workers	Mercurial compounds	Periodontitis, osteomyelitis
Photographic workers	Mercurial compounds	Gingivitis
Polishers and blasters	Dust	Abrasion, pigmentation
Stoneworkers	Dust	Abrasion, gingivitis
X-ray technicians	X-rays (radium)	Xerostomia

Reference: SCHOUR, ISAAC, and SARNAT, B. G.: Oral Manifestations of Occupational Origin. *J.A.M.A.,* **120**:1197-1207, December 12, 1942.

LOCAL FACTORS

SYSTEMIC FACTORS

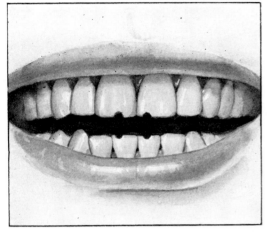

MECHANICAL
Abrasion by tacks

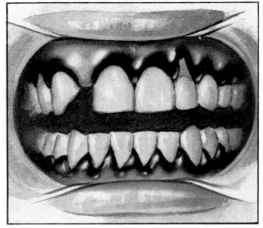

LEAD LINE

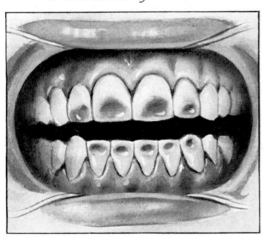

CHEMICAL
Decalcification by acids

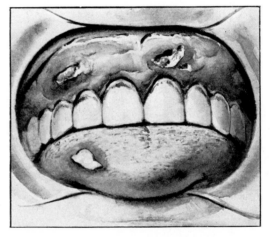

MERCURIAL STOMATITIS

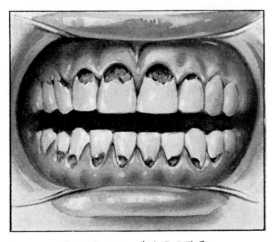

SUGAR CARIES

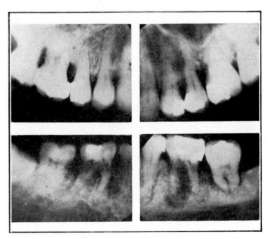

RADIUM POISONING

PLATE 23.

THE FLOOR OF THE MOUTH

A SYSTEMATIC examination of the oral cavity should include the structures lying on the floor of the mouth. This area is readily visible when the tongue is raised. The inferior (ventral) surface of the tongue is smooth and glistening and free of papillae. It is covered with a thin mucous membrane through which some of the underlying structures can be seen (the anterior lingual gland, the large blue lingual vein and the lingual artery and nerve). The floor of the oral cavity (the sublingual region) is in reality the roof of a U-shaped chamber containing the sublingual gland, the anterior part of the submaxillary gland, the lingual and hypoglossal nerves and many blood vessels. This chamber is sometimes called the floor of the mouth.

The sublingual region is extremely vascular. The vessels are superficial and covered by only a thin layer of mucosa. Soluble drugs (nitrites and sulfa and other drugs) placed under the tongue are absorbed into the general circulation rapidly in a manner analogous to absorption from intraperitoneal injections.

Ranula. A retention cyst of the glands of the floor of the mouth pushing up the floor of the mouth and giving it the appearance of a frog's belly.

Ludwig's Angina. A virulent extensive phlegmonous process starting in the chamber of the floor of the mouth. It is characterized by severe involvement of the cervical cellular tissue (cellulitis), which feels hard and board-like, and by a profound toxemia. It is most frequently caused by direct extension of a virulent (usually streptococcic) periapical infection into the floor of the mouth. Extension of the infection from the confines of the floor of the mouth is usually fatal. Early treatment with the sulfa drugs has markedly reduced the mortality.

Reference: CALLANDER, C. L.: Surgical Anatomy. Philadelphia: W. B. Saunders Co., 1939.

THE FLOOR OF THE MOUTH

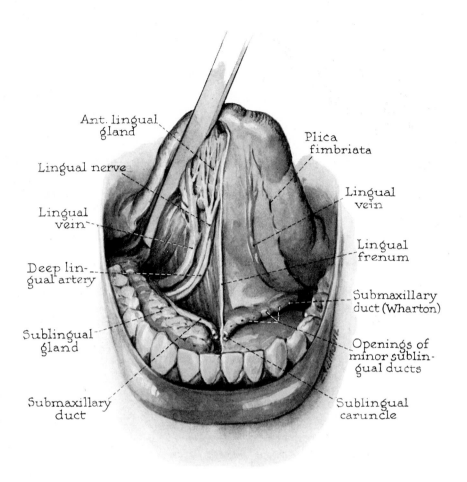

Ant. lingual gland

Plica fimbriata

Lingual nerve

Lingual vein

Lingual vein

Lingual frenum

Deep lingual artery

Submaxillary duct (Wharton)

Sublingual gland

Openings of minor sublingual ducts

Submaxillary duct

Sublingual caruncle

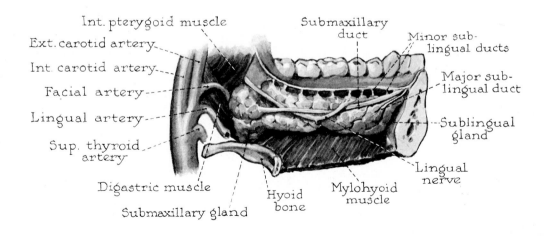

Int. pterygoid muscle

Submaxillary duct

Ext. carotid artery

Minor sublingual ducts

Int. carotid artery

Major sublingual duct

Facial artery

Lingual artery

Sublingual gland

Sup. thyroid artery

Lingual nerve

Digastric muscle

Hyoid bone

Mylohyoid muscle

Submaxillary gland

PLATE 24.

THE SALIVARY GLANDS

SALIVARY glands are found throughout the oral cavity except on the alveolar process, in the anterior portion of the palate and at the occlusal level of the cheek. In certain areas these glands are grouped into large-sized major glands.

Glands	Location	Excretory Ducts	Type	Secretion	
				Function	Stimulus
Parotid	On lateral aspect of mandibular ramus in front of ear and in retro-mandibular fossa; largest gland	Stenson's duct; opens on a teat-like projection opposite upper second molar	Almost entirely serous (ptyalin); clear and watery secretion	Cleansing; dissolving; digestive	Sour (Lemon)
Submaxillary	On inner aspect of mandible reaching to hyoid bone; intermediate gland	Wharton's duct; opens on sublingual caruncle	Mixed; mostly serous; thin at first, later thicker	Lubricative; digestive	?
Sublingual	In floor of mouth next to body of mandible; smallest major gland	Bartholin's duct; opens on sublingual caruncle; several accessory Rivinian ducts open on plica sublingualis	Mostly mucous (mucilaginous and ropey)	Lubricative	Bland substances (milk, bread)
Minor Glands Labial Buccal Palatal Lingual	 Lips Cheeks Palate Tongue		 Mucous and serous Mucous and serous Mucous Mucous and serous		

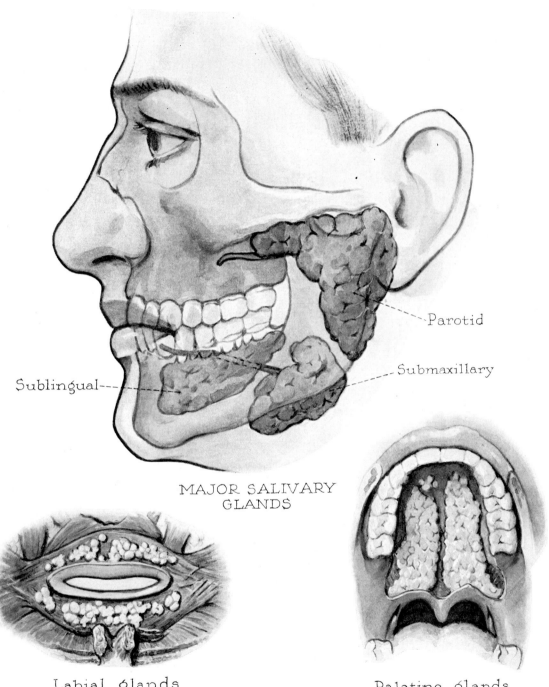

MAJOR SALIVARY
GLANDS

Parotid

Submaxillary

Sublingual

Labial glands
(Viewed from inside)

Palatine glands

MINOR SALIVARY GLANDS

PLATE 25.

THE TONSILS

(WALDEYER'S RING)

WALDEYER'S ring is a ring of lymphoid tissue surrounding the entrance to the pharynx and localized in some areas to form definite anatomic structures that are readily visible from the mouth :

1. Palatine (Faucial) tonsils, between the anterior and posterior pillars.
2. Pharyngeal tonsils, on the roof of the nasopharynx.
3. Lingual tonsils, in the base of the tongue.
4. Small discrete lymph follicles, on the posterior oropharyngeal wall.

Function. Waldeyer's ring of lymphoid tissue is in intimate relation with the overlying epithelium and serves as a second line of defense and a barrier against bacterial invasion.

Clinical Considerations. *Changes with Age:* All lymphoid tissue, particularly Waldeyer's ring, is normally well developed in children. After puberty, atrophy and recession occur so that, in the adult, the tonsils are measurably reduced in size.

Inflammation: Because of its exposed position and its function, the lymphoid tissue is commonly and normally in a state of inflammation. When the body is threatened with invasion, or the integrity of the epithelium is destroyed, the tissue becomes acutely inflamed. In the absence of a distinct pathologic lesion, it cannot be said with certainty that a given tonsil is diseased.

The crypts in the faucial tonsils often become filled with debris and materia alba (as do the interproximal areas between the teeth). This has often been mistaken for pus and tonsillectomy has been advised.

THE TONSILS

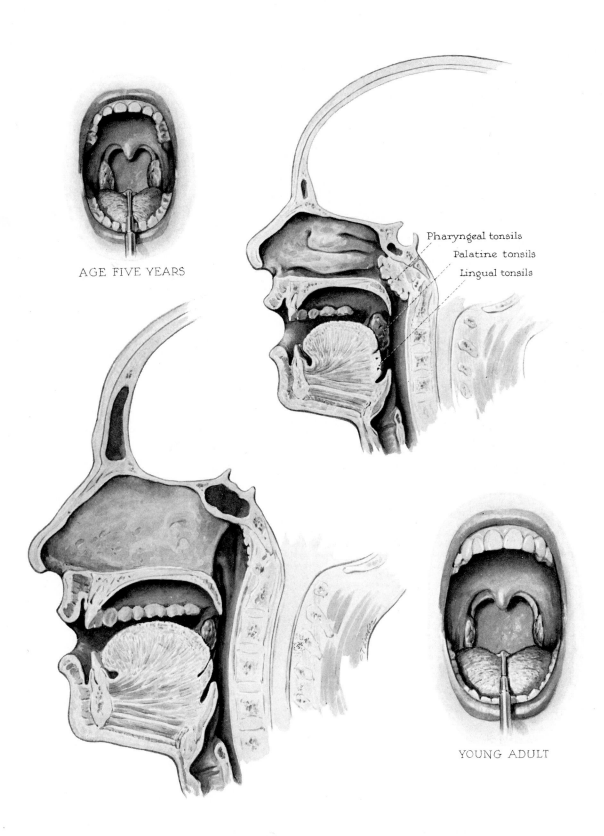

AGE FIVE YEARS

Pharyngeal tonsils
Palatine tonsils
Lingual tonsils

YOUNG ADULT

PLATE 26.

COMMON AILMENTS OF THE THROAT

THE state of health of the throat must be considered by the dentist when examining and treating the oral cavity. A thorough understanding of the "normal" throat can be acquired only by routine examination of the throats of many persons. Oral infections readily spread to the pharynx. Infections of the throat may also extend into the mouth.

Follicular Tonsillitis. Acute inflammation of the lymphoid tissue and its surrounding area followed by swelling of the tonsils and the pillars.

Vincent's Angina. Infection of the pharyngeal tissue and the tonsils by Vincent's organisms and characterized by a marked systemic reaction, injection of the surrounding mucosa and the formation of crater-like ulcerations and a pseudo-membrane. The process may extend to or originate from the gingivae.

Peritonsillar Abscess (Quinsy). Extension of acute tonsillar infection into the peritonsillar tissue. The condition is very painful and may require surgical drainage for relief. The tonsils should be removed after the attack.

Septic Sore Throat. Infection by *Streptococcus hemolyticus.* It is usually milk-borne and epidemic. The throat is very sore and red. The systemic reaction is usually severe and accompanied by fever.

Reference: LEDERER, F. L., and HOLLENDER, A. R.: Textbook of Ear, Nose and Throat. Philadelphia: F. A. Davis Co., 1942.

COMMON AILMENTS OF THE THROAT

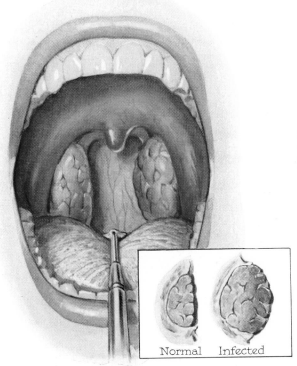

FOLLICULAR TONSILLITIS

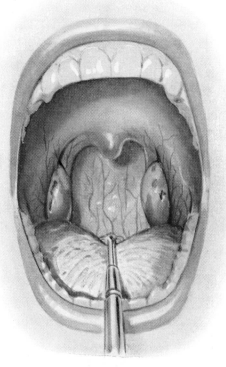

VINCENT'S ANGINA

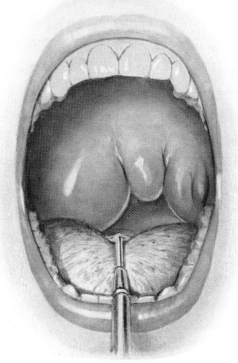

PERITONSILLAR ABSCESS (QUINSY)

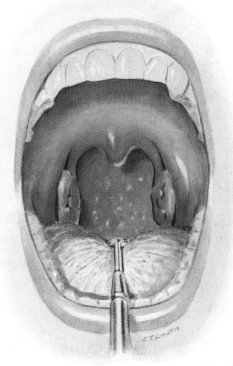

SEPTIC SORE THROAT (STREPTOCOCCUS)

PLATE 27.

THE PARANASAL SINUSES

THE paranasal sinuses are air cavities in the bones above and at each side of the nasal cavities.

The sinuses are connected with the nasal cavities by openings or channels so that the mucous membrane of the sinuses is continuous with that of the nose. In this manner, ventilation and drainage of the sinuses are made possible.

The sinuses, which are named after the bones which they pneumatize, consist of two groups:

Anterior group, opening into the middle meatus:
Maxillary sinus (antrum).
Frontal sinus.
Anterior ethmoid cells.

Posterior group:
Sphenoidal sinus, opening into the spheno-ethmoidal recess.
Posterior ethmoid cells, opening into the superior meatus.

Functions. The air spaces:

(1) reduce the weight of the skull;

(2) give resonance to the voice (note the nasal tone in persons with colds and mouth breathers) and

(3) act as reserve chambers to warm the respired air. During inspiration, the suction through the nasal cavity draws some warmed air from the sinuses.

Clinical Considerations. The roots of the upper bicuspids and molars lie in proximity to the floor of the maxillary sinus and at best are separated by a very thin layer of spongy bone. Often they are separated by no bone at all, so that the root ends are covered by the mucous membrane of the sinus. Because of this anatomic relationship, periapical infections in the upper posterior teeth may spread rapidly to the maxillary sinus. The extraction of these teeth must also be carried out with care lest a traumatic sinusitis result or a root be pushed into the antrum.

Disease of the sinuses may result from extension of nasal disease (head colds), from any interference with physiologic function of the nasal cavity or its lining or from extension of dentogenic infections.

The symptoms of sinus infection are: pain over the sinuses, headache, blocked nose with perhaps nasal discharge and a slight fever. Those resulting from dentogenic infection are characterized by a foul-smelling discharge. Maxillary sinusitis is frequently accompanied by tenderness of some or all of the upper teeth.

Reference: NEIRERT, H.: Surgery of Nose and Sinuses; in Kernan's Surgery of Nose and Throat. New York: Thomas Nelson & Sons, 1942.

THE PARANASAL SINUSES

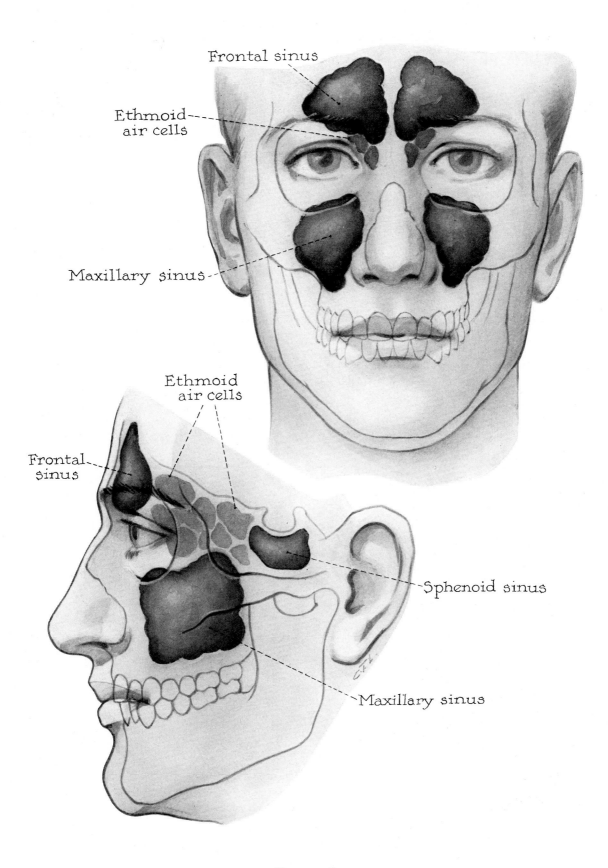

Frontal sinus

Ethmoid air cells

Maxillary sinus

Ethmoid air cells

Frontal sinus

Sphenoid sinus

Maxillary sinus

PLATE 28.

EFFECTS OF MOUTH BREATHING

NASAL breathing is essential to the normal well-being of the body. Breathing through the nose permits the air to be warmed, moistened and cleansed before it reaches the lungs.

In mouth breathers, the preparation of the air for the lungs is lacking so that the child becomes susceptible to upper respiratory infections. In addition, the dental apparatus and the delicate, growing bony structures of the face are so affected that a typical "adenoid" facies results.

Facial Changes ("Adenoid" Facies). The face becomes markedly elongated and narrowed because of dropping of the mandible into an open position and because of the constriction of the upper arches and palate. The nostrils become narrowed and pinched from disuse. The expression becomes dull and drawn.

Etiology. Mouth breathing may result from (1) nasal obstruction, by enlargement of the pharyngeal tonsils or (2) habit. It occurs most frequently in long-faced (dolichofacial), tall slender persons (ectomorphs) in whom the pharyngeal space is normally long, but very narrow.

Treatment. Surgical removal of the obstruction. Muscle exercises to strengthen the lips and to maintain closure. Orthodontic treatment is frequently necessary to make the closed-mouth position comfortable.

In the child whose normal nasal function is obstructed so that he is obliged to breathe through his mouth, the following changes occur:

1. **The lips** become slack and stay open so that the upper lip is shortened and elevated from over the upper incisors, while the lower lip becomes heavy and everted and usually lies beneath and behind the upper incisors instead of over them. The molding action of the lips on the upper incisors is thus lost, a protrusion of these teeth, with spacing, resulting.

2. **The gingivae** frequently are hypertrophied and inflamed in the cuspid-to-cuspid region.

3. **The tongue** is kept suspended between the arches or on the floor of the mouth instead of on the roof, so that the molding action of the tongue is lost to the upper buccal segments, leaving them unapposed to the action of the buccal musculature.

4. **The maxillary arch** and the maxillae become V-shaped owing to contraction of the buccal segments and protrusion of the anterior teeth. **The palate** is high.

5. **The mandible** is retruded and hangs open in a slack manner.

6. **The maxillary sinuses** and **nasal cavity** frequently become narrowed as the upper arch is contracted, with further narrowing of the face.

7. **The turbinates** become swollen and engorged.

8. **The nasal mucosa** becomes atrophic from disuse, and the alae nasi become narrowed and pinched. The speech acquires a "nasal" tone. The bacteriostatic action of the nasal secretions is lost, and a pathway is permitted whereby disease, particularly virus infections, may enter. *The sense of smell* is dulled, and with it, taste sensations and the appetite.

9. **The lymphoid tissues** become hyperplastic from venous stasis and the impact of cold, dust-laden air. Occasionally, such hyperplasia of the adenoids will occlude the opening of the eustachian tube and result in defective hearing.

Reference: PROETZ, A. W.: Essays on Applied Physiology of Nose. St. Louis: Annals Publishing Co., 1941.

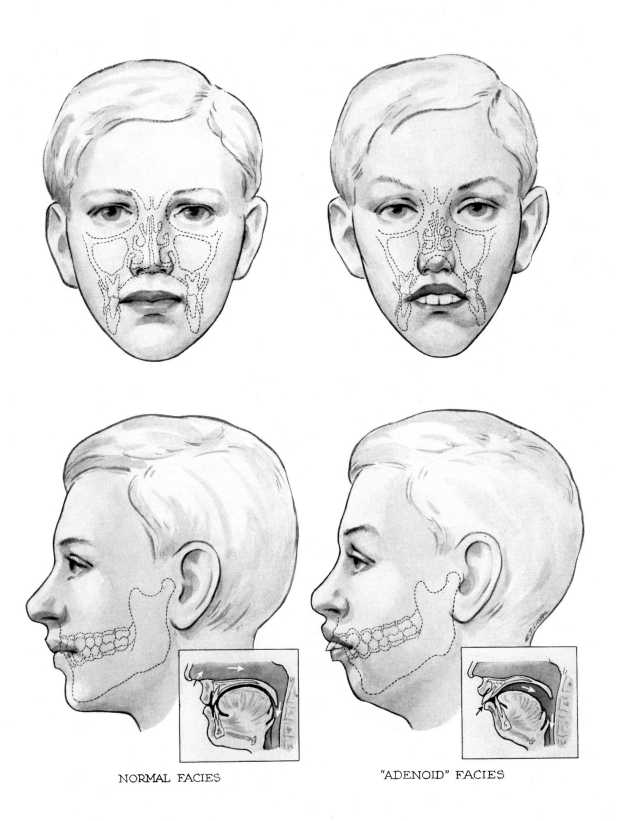

NORMAL FACIES   "ADENOID" FACIES

PLATE 29.

FRONTAL AND HORIZONTAL SECTIONS THROUGH THE FACE

A KNOWLEDGE of the anatomic relationships of the intra-oral and circum-oral structures is essential to diagnosis, prevention and therapy in dental practice.

The serious complications that may follow periapical infections can often be controlled or prevented by an understanding of the anatomic basis for the spread of such infections. Heat (or counterirritation) is effective in controlling the spread of dental infections provided it is applied at the right point and in harmony with the anatomic characteristics of the region involved.

Periapical infection should be localized so that the area can open and drain into the vestibule of the mouth. The majority of periapical infections point into the oral cavity since the warm and moist environment invites localization. Nature can be aided by increasing the intra-oral heat by means of hot mouth washes or counterirritants. Extra-oral heat may favor the spread of the periapical infection into the cheek, leading to perforation of the skin and a disfiguring scar.

Periapical infections, when not localized, may spread by the following routes:

1. Direct extension:

   (a) Invasion and infection of the jaw-bone (osteomyelitis).
   (b) Invasion and infection of adjacent structures:

      Upper posterior teeth—maxillary sinus infection.
      Upper cuspid and bicuspid teeth—subperiosteally to the orbit.
      Upper anterior teeth—floor of nose, ethmoiditis.
      Lower posterior teeth—floor of mouth and parapharyngeal space infections.
      Lower anterior teeth—floor of mouth infections.

2. Extension along fascial planes:

   Fascial planes are potential spaces which are ideal sites for the collection of pus and the development of cellulitis. The following spaces are most commonly involved:

   Cheek: Masticator, temporal and parotid spaces.
   Neck: Floor of mouth (sublingual space), submaxillary space and the carotid sheath.
   Pharynx: Pharyngomaxillary (parapharyngeal) space.

3. Extension via the lymphatics:

   The lymphatics of the periodontal structures drain into the submaxillary lymph glands, except those from the lower anterior region, which drain into the submental lymph glands. If the infection is virulent, cellulitis may result.

4. Spread via the venous system:

   (a) Periapical infections of the upper anterior teeth (particularly in children) may enter into the lip or floor of the nose and spread along the anterior facial vein to the cavernous sinus. Infections in the nasal cavity may ascend to the ethmoid air cells.

   (b) Focal infection (periapical infection) may enter into the general circulation and become localized in distant structures that are traumatized or of weak resistance.

Reference: THOMA, K. H.: Oral Diagnosis. Ed. 2. Philadelphia: W. B. Saunders and Co., 1943.

FRONTAL SECTION THROUGH THE FACE

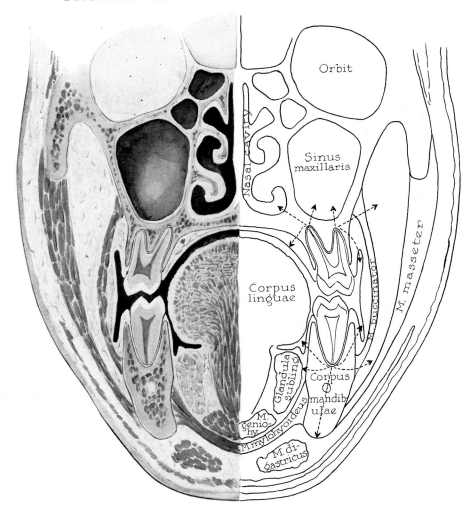

Orbit

Nasal cavity

Sinus maxillaris

M. masseter

M. buccinator

Corpus linguae

Glandula subling

Corpus mandibulae

M. geniohy

M. mylohyoideus

M. digastricus

HORIZONTAL SECTION THROUGH THE FACE

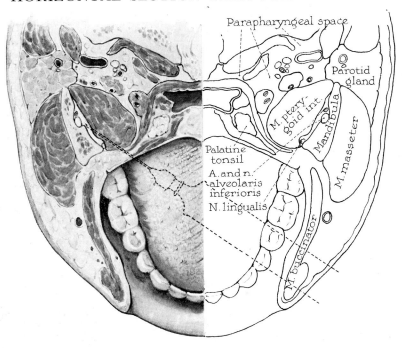

Parapharyngeal space

Parotid gland

M. ptery-goid int.

Mandibula

M. masseter

Palatine tonsil

A. and n. alveolaris inferioris

N. lingualis

M. buccinator

PLATE 30.

ARTERIES OF THE HEAD

THE head receives its arterial blood supply from the common carotid artery, which divides below the hyoid bone into the internal and external carotid arteries. The internal carotid artery lies deep and enters the carotid canal to supply the brain, the eye and the adjacent areas.

The external carotid (1) artery, which is more superficial, supplies the rest of the head, including the dental apparatus. The branches of the external carotid artery are named according to the area that they supply. The important branches are given off in the following order:

Superior thyroid artery (runs downward to supply the thyroid gland).

Lingual artery (2) (enters deep in the neck to supply the tongue).

External maxillary artery (3) (crosses the lower border of the mandible at the mandibular notch to supply the face).

Occipital artery (runs posteriorly and exits behind the mastoid process to supply the occipital area).

At the level of the mandibular condyle, the external carotid splits into two branches:

Internal maxillary artery (entering deep behind the neck of the condyle).

Superficial temporal artery (4) (crosses the zygomatic arch and supplies most of the scalp).

Clinical Considerations. In order to stop hemorrhage as quickly as possible after traumatic injury to the face, one must seek a point where the artery can be reached by digital pressure. A point where the artery crosses a bony structure is desirable, since the digital pressure is then over a bony, non-yielding area and the artery is tightly compressed between the bone and the thumb. Such compression may lessen bleeding sufficiently to save a life.

The external maxillary artery supplies most of the face and can be compressed at the point (3) where it curves over the inferior border of the mandible at the mandibular notch to continue as the external facial artery. The mandibular notch and the vessels can easily be felt with the thumb.

Most of the scalp is supplied by the superficial temporal artery, which can easily be compressed as it crosses the zygomatic arch just in front of the ear.

Reference: Manual of Standard Practice of Plastic and Maxillofacial Surgery, Military Surgical Manuals, National Research Council, 1942, pp. 264-265.

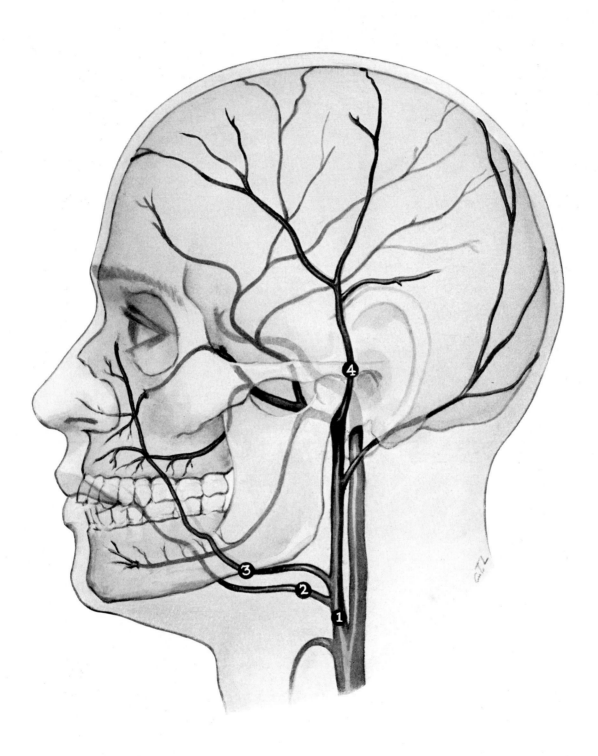

PLATE 31.

VEINS OF THE HEAD

A KNOWLEDGE of the venous blood supply and its flow is essential to an understanding of the routes whereby blood-borne infections may lead to serious and even fatal complications.

Cavernous sinus thrombosis may be of dental origin. Two main routes of infection are possible:

1. **The Facial or External Route.** This route consists of a large, open system of veins leading directly to the cavernous sinus. The infection, therefore, spreads very rapidly. The course is fulminating and of short duration, and ends with a classic picture of a cavernous sinus thrombosis.

Infections of the upper anterior teeth, the upper lip and alae of the nose are liable to enter the anterior facial vein via the labial veins. The infection then continues upward to the inner canthus of the eye, where it enters the angular and nasofrontal veins. The infection then generally enters the superior ophthalmic vein, causing a proptosis of the eye (see inset), and then passes through the superior orbital fissure and enters directly into the anterior end of the cavernous sinus.

About 4 per cent of the fatal cases of thrombosis of the cavernous sinus in children are of dental origin. The dangers of spreading a mild infection of the upper lip or in the nose by "squeezing" or "picking" are well known to the physician. What is generally less well appreciated is that periapical infection of the upper anterior teeth may follow the same route and similarly cause a cavernous sinus infection.

2. **The Pterygoid or Internal Route.** This route runs through a complicated network of small veins and leads to the cavernous sinus only through many small twisting by-passes. The infection spreads in a slow and in a retrograde manner. Its worst feature is the frequent lack of obvious symptoms until the cavernous sinus is actually infected.

Infections of the posterior teeth, particularly the lower molars, may reach the pterygoid plexus (a) directly from the alveolar network, (b) indirectly from the upper posterior teeth via the posterior facial and internal maxillary veins or (c) from the upper anterior teeth via the anterior facial and deep facial veins. Once in the pterygoid plexus, the infection travels very slowly upward and may reach the cavernous sinus (a) directly via a few small veins or (b) indirectly via the larger inferior ophthalmic vein.

Arrows indicate the direction of the spread of the infection.

Reference: CHILDS, H. G., and COURVILLE, C. B.: Thrombosis of Cavernous Sinus Secondary to Dental Infection. *Am. J. Orthodontics,* 28:367, June; 402, July; 458, August; 515, September 1942.

VEINS OF THE HEAD

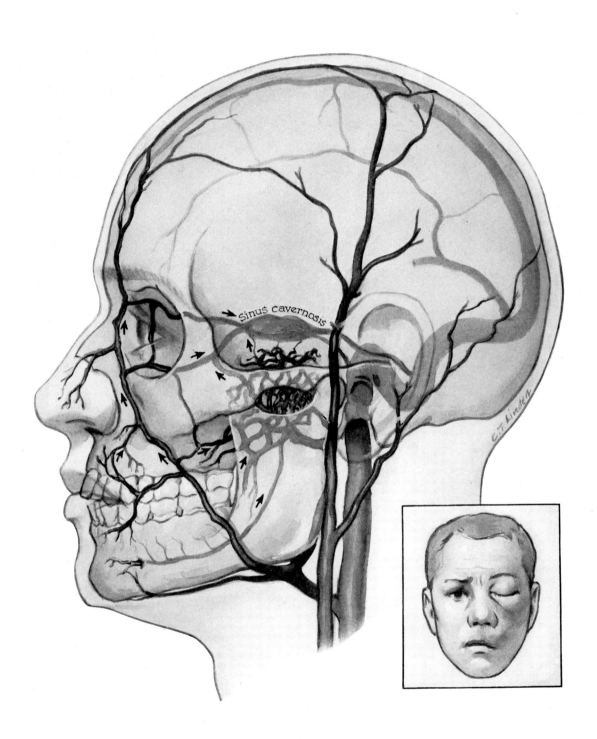

Sinus cavernosis

PLATE 32.

THE TRIGEMINAL NERVE

THE fifth cranial nerve is mainly responsible for the cutaneous supply of the face and scalp. In addition, it provides the motor-innervation for the muscles of mastication. The major portion is sensory and gives rise to three divisions: ophthalmic, maxillary and mandibular.

An accurate knowledge of the topographic anatomy of the sensory branches of the trigeminal nerve, particularly of the location of their bony entrances and exits, is essential to the successful application of block anesthesia.

	Internal Branches (Visceral)	Intermediary Branches (Anterior)	External Branches (Lateral)
Div. I. (Ophthalmic)	N. nasociliaris	N. frontalis (N. supraorbitalis)	N. lacrimalis
Div. II. (Maxillary)	N. sphenopalatini (rami nasales and N. palatini)	N. infraorbitalis	N. zygomaticus
Div. III. (Mandibular)	N. buccinatorius N. lingualis	N. alveolaris inferioris (N. mentalis)	N. auriculo-temporalis

Nevi (or congenital hemangiomas) tend to follow very closely the distribution of the three divisions of the trigeminal nerve and demarcate the areas of supply as if by "vital staining." (See inset.)

Reference: SICHER, HARRY, and TANDLER, J.: Anatomie für Zahnärzte, 1928.

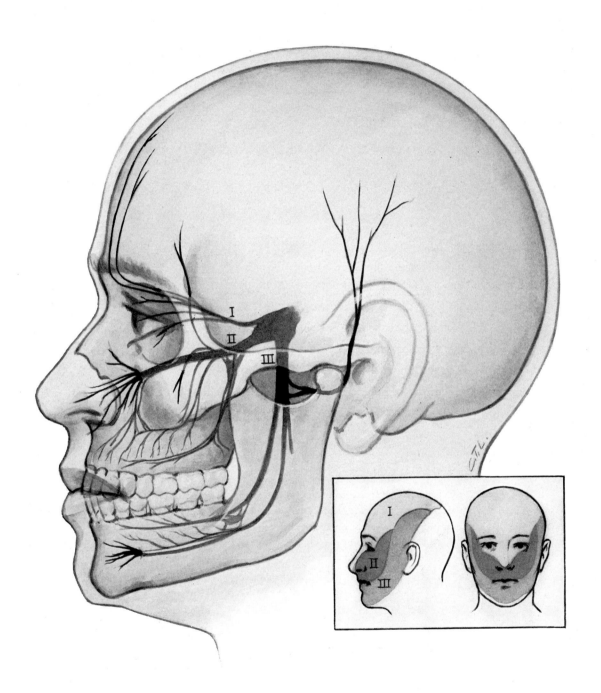

PLATE 33.

ANATOMY OF THE TEMPOROMANDIBULAR JOINT

THE anatomy of the temporomandibular joint is of special importance to the dentist since it is by this joint that the denture is articulated. Disturbances in the temporomandibular articulation usually result in disturbances of the occlusion.

The mandible, the only movable bone in the face, is held in position by the muscles of mastication and is attached to the cranium by the ligaments of the joint.

The condylar head of the mandible lies in the glenoid fossa of the temporal bone and is separated from it by the meniscus. When the jaw and the teeth are at physiologic rest, the condylar head touches the anterior part (articular portion) of the fossa.

The Capsular Ligament surrounds the joint completely and is attached to the margins of the articulating surfaces of the temporal bone (mandibular fossa and articular fossa) and to the neck of the condyle. (Not labeled in Plate 34.)

Clinical Considerations: The facial nerve (N. VII) crosses below the mandibular neck. Care must be taken during surgical procedures in this area lest the nerve be injured and a facial paralysis result. Injuries to the seventh nerve tend to be permanent.

Reference: SHAPIRO, H. H.: Applied Anatomy of Head and Neck. Philadelphia: J. B. Lippincott Co., 1943.

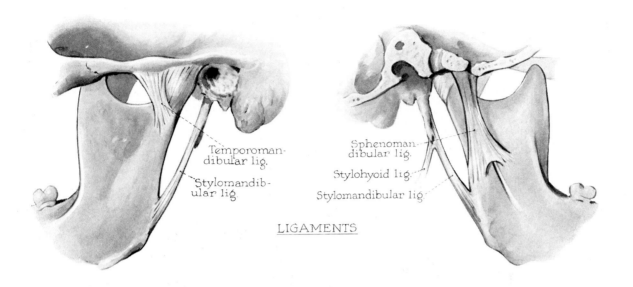

Temporoman-
dibular lig.

Stylomandib-
ular lig.

Sphenoman-
dibular lig.

Stylohyoid lig.

Stylomandibular lig.

LIGAMENTS

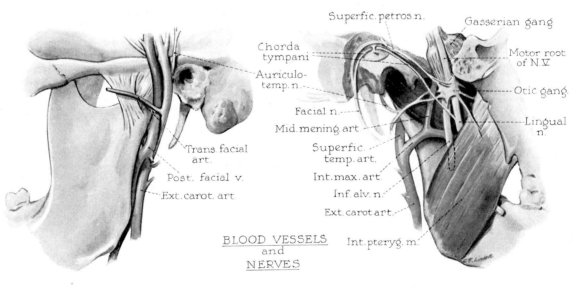

Superfic. petros. n.

Gasserian gang

Chorda
tympani

Motor root
of N.V

Auriculo-
temp. n.

Otic gang.

Facial n.

Lingual
n.

Mid. mening. art.

Superfic.
temp. art.

Int. max. art.

Inf. alv. n.

Ext. carot. art.

Trans. facial
art.

Post. facial v.

Ext. carot. art.

BLOOD VESSELS
and
NERVES

Int. pteryg. m.

LATERAL VIEW

MEDIAL VIEW

PLATE 34.

ACTION OF THE TEMPOROMANDIBULAR JOINT

THE temporomandibular joint is a compound multiaxial joint so constructed as to permit different types of movement of the mandible and different degrees of mouth opening. This is made possible by the presence of the meniscus, which divides the joint into an upper and a lower compartment.

Hinge Action. The first phase in mouth opening is a simple hinge action. The lower half of the joint only is used, the condyle head rotating around a point on the under surface of the meniscus. The body of the mandible drops almost passively downward and backward.

Gliding Action. The second phase involves the upper compartment of the joint and consists of a gliding of the condylar head, the meniscus and the lower compartment of the joint forward and downward over the eminentia articularis of the zygomatic process of the temporal bone. This occurs alone during protrusion and lateral movements of the mandible and in combination with the hinge action during the forced wider opening of the mouth.

A wide opening of the mouth would be impossible with a simple hinge movement since the posterior surface of the ramus would compress the soft tissues between the mandible and the mastoid process. The gliding action brings the ramus forward and also downward so that the hinge action can continue.

During rotation, the point at which the nerves and blood vessels enter the mandible is at relative rest so that these structures are not injured by stretching.

Reference: BRODIE, A. G.: The Temporomandibular Joint. *Illinois D. J.*, 8:2-12, January 1939.

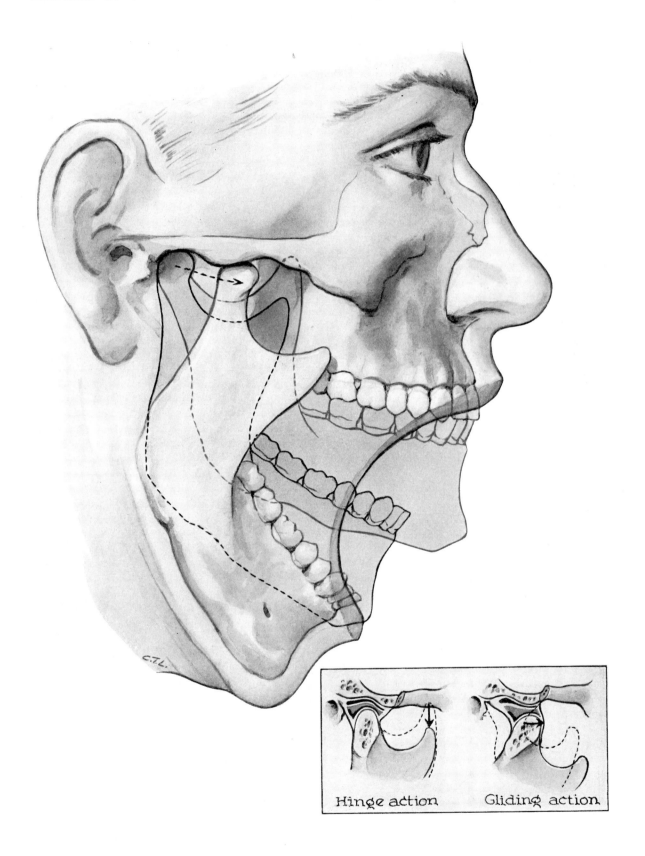

Hinge action   Gliding action

PLATE 35.

ABNORMAL OPENINGS OF THE MOUTH

AN abnormal amount of mouth opening results when the condylar head travels too far over the articular eminence. This displacement may be partial and self-reducing (subluxation) or complete, in which case self-reduction is not possible (dislocation).

Dislocation. Dislocation may result from an excessive opening of the mouth during yawning, prolonged dental operations (particularly during tooth extraction) or efforts to force a very large bolus of food into the mouth. The condylar head is forced over the articular eminence and into the zygomatic fossa. The capsular ligaments are stretched, but generally are not torn. The condylar head is kept from returning to the glenoid fossa by the articular eminence. Immediately after dislocation, trismus of the muscles of mastication tends to freeze the dislocation into an open-mouth position, but, after a time, the muscles may relax and permit a hinge movement of the condylar head with the mandible in the protruded position. Speech is difficult.

Treatment is by manual reduction. It may be necessary to anesthetize the patient to relax the muscles of mastication. In habitual dislocations, the injection of the joint is indicated.

Subluxation (Partial Dislocation). Some persons frequently open the mouth very wide, forcing the condylar head to jump to the very tip of the articulated eminence. Self-reduction occurs upon closing the mouth. In most cases, the habitual excessive opening of the mouth causes the capsular ligaments to become stretched beyond their normal limits and the meniscus to become displaced. In such cases, a characteristic clicking or cracking noise is heard during mouth opening.

Habitual subluxation can be treated by Schultz's method of injecting a fibrosing agent (5 per cent solution of sodium psylliate) into the joint cavity and thus limiting the gliding action of the joint.

Reference: SCHULTZ, LOUIS W.: Curative Treatment for Subluxation of Temporomandibular Joint. *J.A.D.A.,* 12:671, June 1925.

ABNORMAL OPENINGS OF THE MOUTH

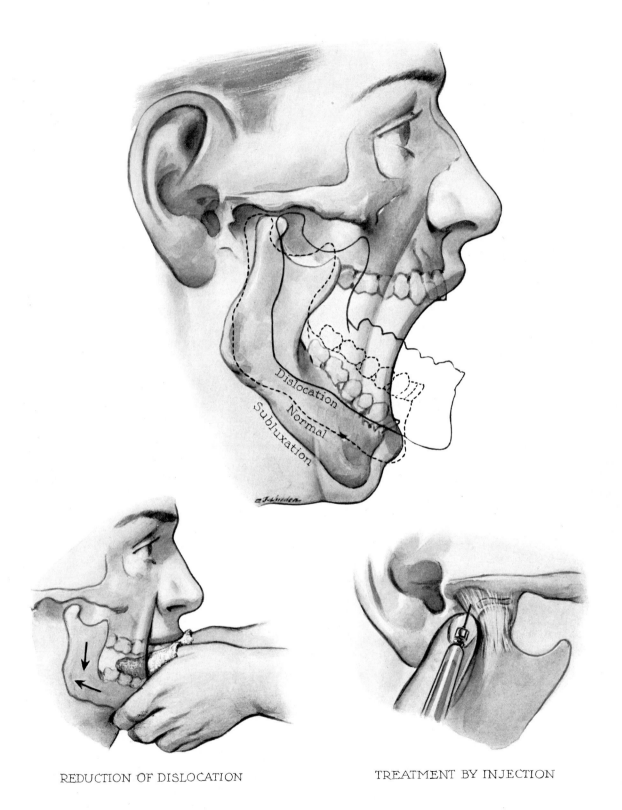

REDUCTION OF DISLOCATION   TREATMENT BY INJECTION

PLATE 36.

ABNORMAL CLOSURE OF THE TEMPOROMANDIBULAR JOINT

OVERCLOSURE of the temporomandibular joint may occur during function when the intermaxillary vertical dimension is less than it should be because of excessive occlusal wear, loss of the posterior teeth or the wearing of improperly made artificial dentures. The overclosure results from the powerful pull of the masseter and internal pterygoid muscles during mastication. During physiologic rest, this pressure is relieved.

It has been suggested that overclosure leads to perforation of the meniscus and the bone of the floor of the fossa, causing pain in the temporal region and deafness. To overcome these conditions, bite-raising procedures have been instituted. Recent investigations show that such conditions are rare and that opening of the bite to relieve deafness is not indicated unless proper audiometric tests rule out other possible causes.

Reference: SHAPIRO, H. H., and TRUEX, R. C.: Temporomandibular Joint and Auditory Function. *J.A.D.A.,* 30:1147, August 1, 1943.

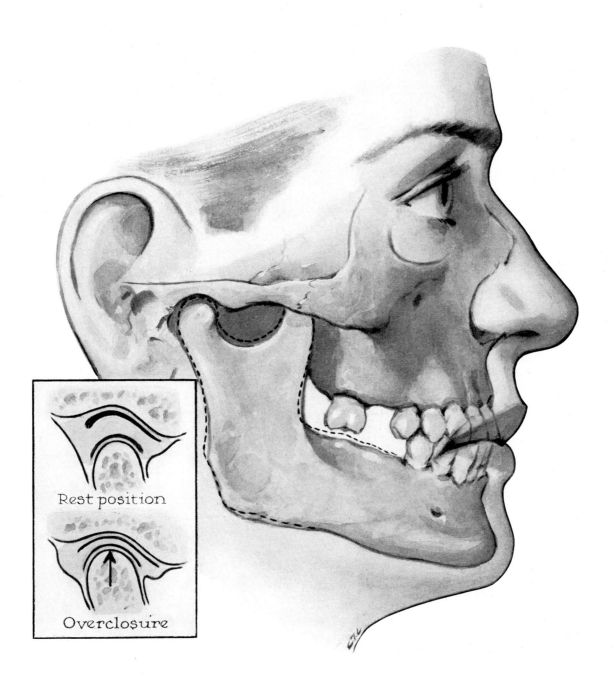

Rest position

Overclosure

PLATE 37.

DEVIATION OF THE MIDLINE IN MOUTH OPENING

DEVIATION of the midline in mouth opening indicates a unilateral partial ankylosis by fibrosis of the temporomandibular joint (or a paralysis of the motor root of the fifth nerve). A partial ankylosis results in loss of the gliding action, while paralysis inhibits the action of the external pterygoid muscle, with the same result. If the excursion is lost on one side for either reason, the chin point will deviate toward the affected side during wide opening.

Bilateral partial ankylosis (loss of gliding movement, but normal hinge action in both joints) results in restricted mouth opening, but no midline deviation. Complete ankylosis (bony), unilateral or bilateral, results in marked restriction of mouth opening.

Reference: BRODIE, A. G.: Differential Diagnosis of Joint Conditions in Orthodontia. *Angle Orthodontist,* 4:160-170, 1934.

DEVIATION OF THE MIDLINE IN MOUTH OPENING

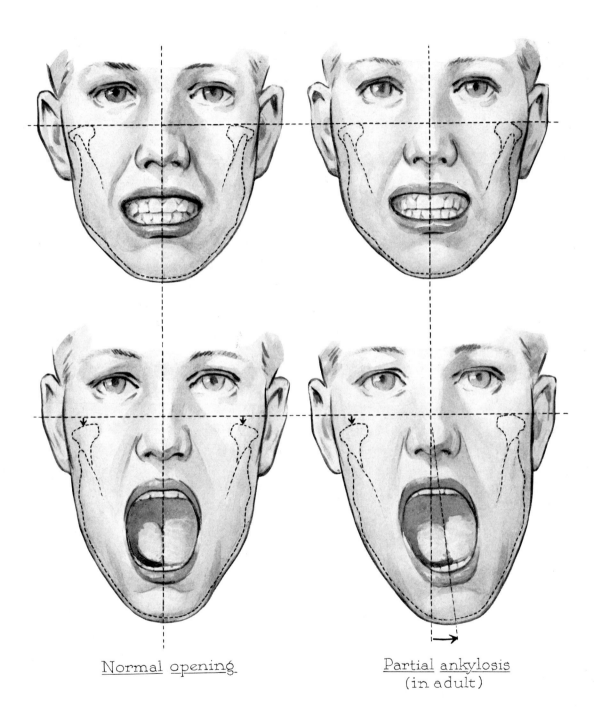

Normal opening

Partial ankylosis
(in adult)

PLATE 38.

FACIAL ASYMMETRY

FACIAL asymmetry resulting from injury to the growing cartilage on the condylar head is fairly common. Traumatic injuries may occur during birth from the placing of obstetrical forceps over the area, or may result from blows on the chin during infancy and childhood.

The condylar head is the site of most active bone growth in the mandible. This growth center is an area of adjustment whereby mandibular growth is synchronized with that of the maxilla. If this center is disturbed, a disharmony between the growth of the mandible and maxilla results. Since the condylar head grows under the influence of the pressure forces caused by mastication, it grows by endochondral bone formation.

Traumatic injury to the growing cartilage on the condylar head may result in a failure of that side of the mandible to elongate. The normal side meanwhile continues to grow and pushes the midline toward the affected side. The deformity is exaggerated during mouth opening. The notch on the lower border anteriorly from the angle of the mandible is usually deepened on the affected side. Bilateral injuries to the growing cartilage result in a retrusion of the chin in the midline and a marked distortion of the entire mandible (Vogelgesicht). Bilateral ankylosis also occurs in rheumatoid arthritis during childhood (Still's disease).

Occasionally a facial asymmetry may be caused by the presence of a tumor or foreign object (shrapnel, wood, etc.) inside the glenoid cavity. The onset then is sudden, and clinical diagnosis is simple, since when the mouth is opened, the deviated midline returns to normal.

Reference: THOMPSON, J. R.: Asymmetry of the Face. *J.A.D.A.,* 30:1859-1871, December 1943.

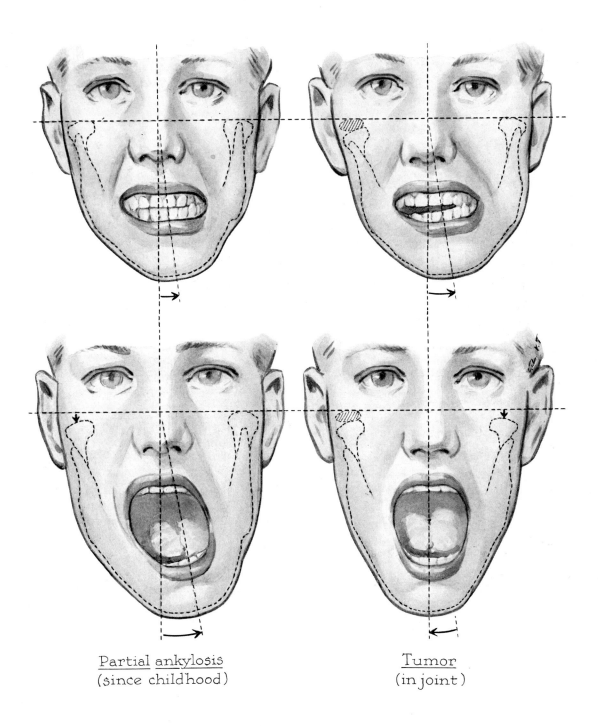

Partial ankylosis
(since childhood)

Tumor
(in joint)

PLATE 39.

THE TEMPORAL MUSCLE

THE temporal muscle arises as a broad fan-shaped expansion from the temporal bone and fascia. It passes under the zygomatic process and is attached to the coronoid process of the mandible. Its tendinous insertion extends down the anterior edge of the ramus and to the temporal crest on the medial surface of the ramus and reaches the level of the occlusal surface of the molar teeth. When the mouth is opened, this extension of the temporal muscle can be readily seen and palpated.

The muscle, when it contracts, pulls the coronoid process upward and backward, snapping the incisors together. Its posterior fibers retract the mandible and are the chief antagonists to the external pterygoid.

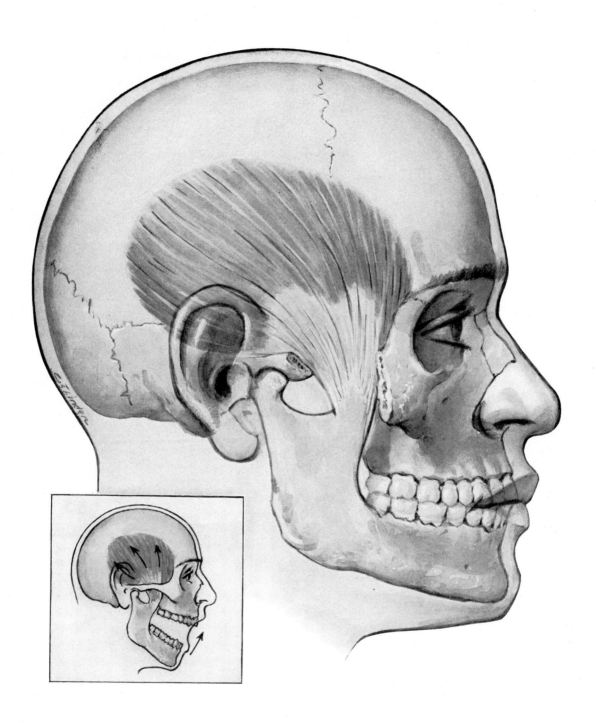

PLATE 40.

THE MASSETER MUSCLE

THE masseter muscle is broad and rhomboidal and covers the greater part of the lateral surface of the ramus and can be readily palpated during function.

The superficial portion arises from the anterior two-thirds of the lower border of the zygomatic process and runs somewhat obliquely downward and backward to insert itself into the lower half of the external surface of the ramus. The deep portion arises from the posterior third of the lower border and internal surface of the zygomatic process and passes nearly vertically downward to insert itself into the upper half of the external surface of the ramus.

The masseter elevates the mandible and brings the molar teeth together for crushing and grinding. It has been called the muscle of determination since it becomes readily visible when the teeth are forcefully clenched.

The masseter is a muscle built for power. Its fibers contract rather slowly but powerfully when stimulated and are specially adapted for the grinding action of the posterior teeth. Its action and position resemble those of the hand on a nutcracker, a position of mechanical advantage for power at the sacrifice of speed. It shows a high development in the herbivora that grind their food thoroughly before swallowing.

The temporal is a snapping muscle, built for speed. Its fibers contract with great rapidity when stimulated and are therefore specially adapted for the snapping action of the anterior teeth. Speed is attained (and power sacrificed) by its position of mechanical advantage in a class three lever; between the fulcrum (the temporomandibular joint) and the object (the anterior teeth). It shows a higher development in the carnivora which snap at and tear their food, but do not grind it before gulping it down. (See inset and Plate 40.)

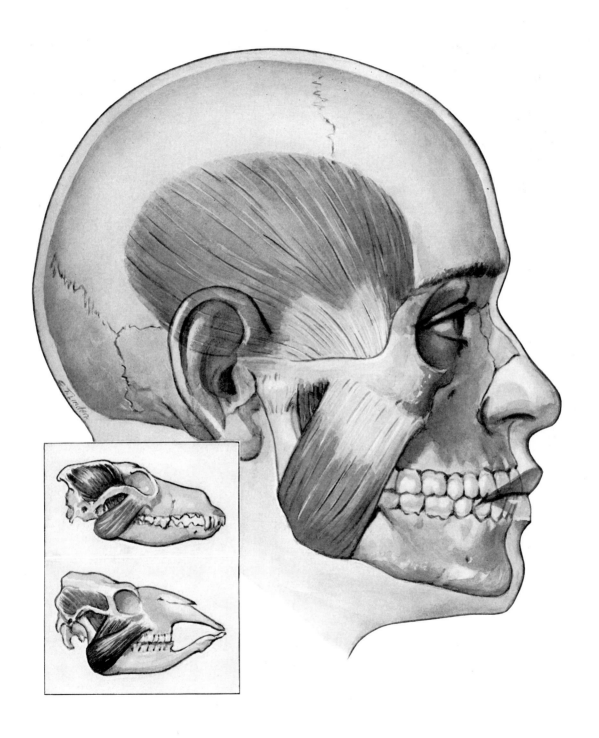

PLATE 41.

THE INTERNAL PTERYGOID MUSCLE

THE internal pterygoid muscle is rhomboidal in shape and arises from the fossa of the pterygoid plate of the sphenoid, for the most part from the medial surface of the lateral pterygoid lamina. Some of its fibers also arise from the maxillary tuberosity and the pyramidal process of the palate bone. It passes downward and backward to insert itself into the internal surface of the ramus and angle of the mandible opposite the region of insertion of the masseter muscle.

The internal pterygoid elevates the mandible and brings the molar teeth together, an action synergistic to that of the masseter on the lateral surface of the ramus.

The internal pterygoid has been called the internal masseter, a term which aptly describes its main function. Both are rhomboidal; have cranial origins and roughly corresponding insertion on the lateral and medial surfaces of the ramus, and both follow a downward and backward course toward the angle of the ramus. Together they form a sling in which the angle of the mandible rests and which straps the ramus to the skull. (See inset.) When acting together, they impart a rotary, grinding action (trituration) to the molar teeth in addition to acting like two overlapping hands on a nutcracker in a forceful crushing action by these teeth. They also act as a natural splint and prevent displacement in fractures of the ramus.

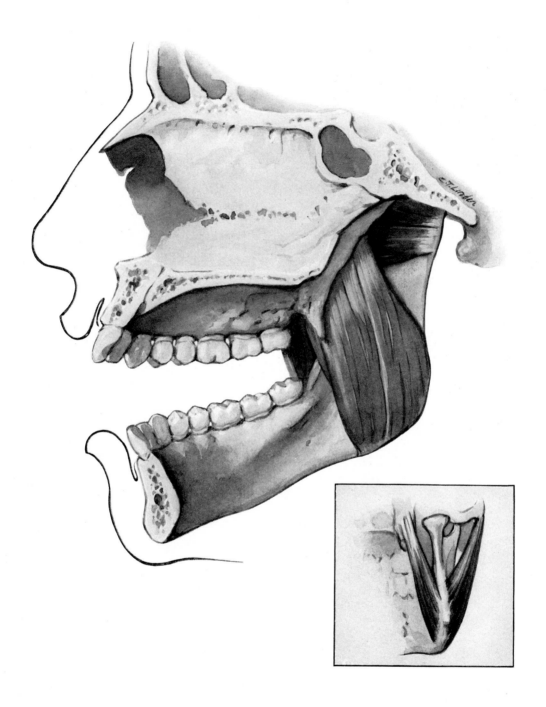

PLATE 42.

THE EXTERNAL PTERYGOID MUSCLE

THE external pterygoid muscle is triangular in shape. It arises by two heads, one from the lateral surface of the external pterygoid plate of the sphenoid and the other from the infratemporal surface of the greater wing of the sphenoid. Its fibers converge as they pass backward and laterally to insert themselves in a pit in front of the neck of the condyle and in the disc of the temporomandibular joint.

The external pterygoids are the opening, protruding and shifting muscles of the jaw. They draw the mandible forward and also rotate it downward. The external ptyerygoids are so positioned that when they contract, they pull the condylar head and the disc forward and so cause a protrusion of the mandible. When they act together, the chin is protruded in the median line. When one muscle alone contracts, the condylar head on that side is displaced forward and the chin is thrust laterally toward the opposite side. (See inset.) When acting alternately and separately, the external pterygoids move the mandible from side to side, as in grinding and chewing.

When the mandible is dropped somewhat, the external pterygoids rotate the mandible downward and backward by rotating the condylar head against a point on the anterior wall of the glenoid fossa near the articular eminence. This action, aided by gravity, opens the mouth as on a hinge. In wider openings of the mouth, the external pterygoids pull the condylar head forward and downward over the articular eminence, while the suprahyoids continue the rotation of the chin downward and backward.

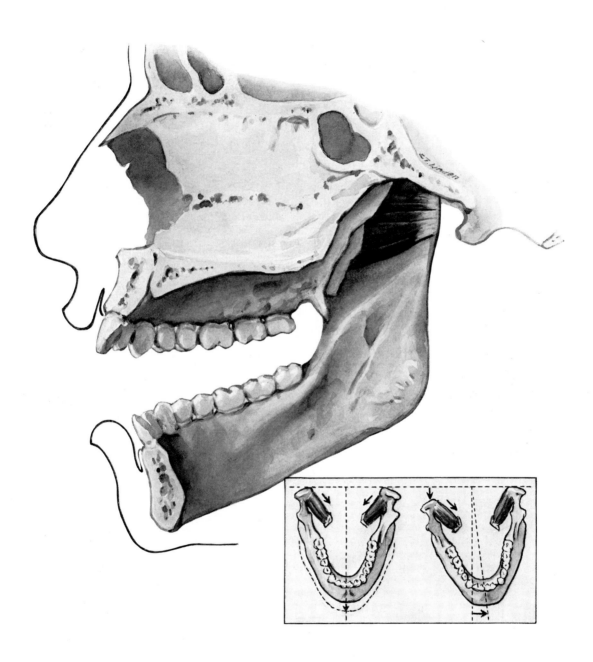

PLATE 43.

MUSCLES OF THE MANDIBLE

THE muscles of the mandible, their origin, insertion and action are important considerations in the analysis of fractures of the mandible. The displacement of the fragments in mandibular fractures is determined by:

1. Direction of the blow.
2. Muscle pull (this is no consideration in maxillary fractures).
3. Direction of line of fracture.
4. Areas of weakness. Direct fractures are those that occur at the point of impact. Indirect fractures frequently occur at a distance from the point of impact in areas of weakness:

(a) Tooth socket (between lamina dura and cementum).
(b) Crypt of unerupted tooth (third molars and cuspids).
(c) Neck of condyle.

The direction of displacement of the fragments when caused entirely by muscle pull may be summed up as follows:

1. *The ramus* has attached to it only the elevator muscles. The fragment is therefore pulled upward.

2. *The body of the mandible* has only depressors attached to it. This fragment is therefore pulled downward.

The body of the mandible has also attached to it the mylohyoid muscle, which has a strong medial pull, and therefore a loosened fragment of the body will also be pulled medially.

3. *The head of the condyle* has only the external pterygoid attached to it. This fragment will therefore be pulled inward and forward.

4. When two or more sets of muscles are attached to any given fragment, the direction of displacement is a resultant of all the forces acting upon it.

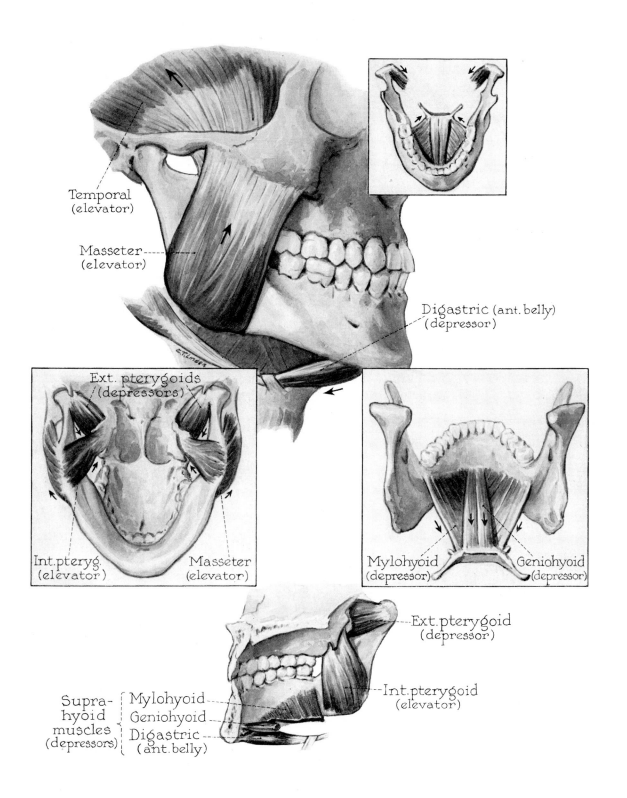

Temporal
(elevator)

Masseter
(elevator)

Digastric (ant. belly)
(depressor)

Ext. pterygoids
(depressors)

Int. pteryg.
(elevator)

Masseter
(elevator)

Mylohyoid
(depressor)

Geniohyoid
(depressor)

Ext. pterygoid
(depressor)

Int. pterygoid
(elevator)

Supra-
hyoid
muscles
(depressors)

Mylohyoid
Geniohyoid
Digastric
(ant. belly)

PLATE 44.

FRACTURES OF THE NECK OF THE CONDYLE

FRACTURES of the neck of the condyle are generally indirect, resulting from frontal or nearly frontal blows on the opposite side. These fractures are fairly common, but not easy to detect without the aid of the roentgenogram.

DISPLACEMENT IN UNILATERAL FRACTURE

(A) **Small Fragment (Head of Condyle):** The condylar head may be rotated inward or pulled forward by the external pterygoid. If the joint capsule is torn, the condylar head may be actually dislocated. (See bottom insets.) The displacement of the condylar head cannot be seen clinically and must be determined roentgenographically.

(B) **Main Body:** The main body is usually displaced toward the injured side, rotating around the uninjured condyle. (See top inset.) A cross-bite usually results. The ramus on the injured side is always pulled up by the elevator muscles.

Opening the mouth causes a marked deviation of the midline toward the injured side. (See also Plate 38.)

DISPLACEMENT IN BILATERAL FRACTURES

(A) **Condylar Heads:** Both may be displaced in any manner shown in the insets.

(B) **Main Body:** Both rami are pulled upward by the elevator muscles, while the chin is pulled down by the depressor muscles. This results in an impaction in the molar region, while the anterior region shows a characteristic open bite.

Reference: BERGER, ADOLPH: Fractures of Mandibular Condyle. *J.A.D.A.,* 30:819-833, June 1, 1943.

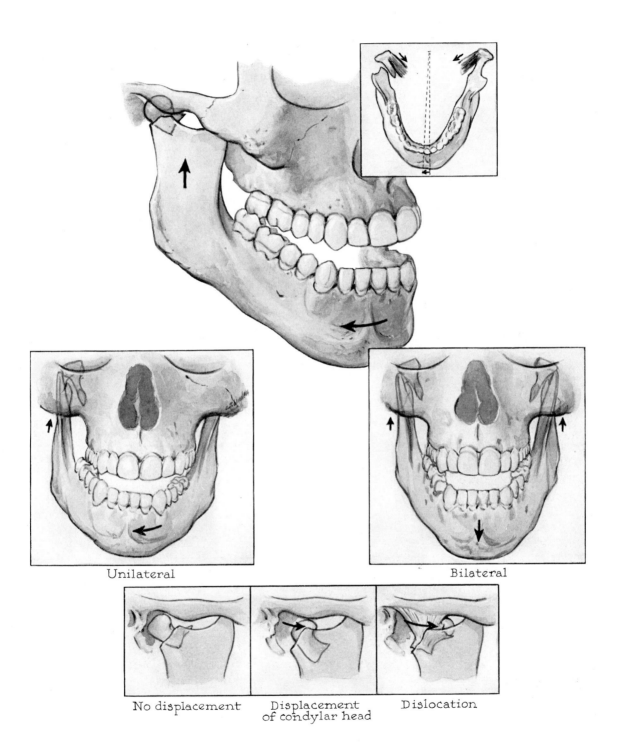

Unilateral

Bilateral

No displacement

Displacement
of condylar head

Dislocation

PLATE 45.

FRACTURES OF THE ANGLE OF THE MANDIBLE

A FRACTURE of the angle of the mandible posterior to the last molar tooth may be caused by a direct blow on the ramus or may be indirect, resulting from a blow on the opposite bicuspid area. The line of fracture usually passes through the crypt of the lower third molar.

The direction of the line of fracture in both the horizontal and the vertical planes is important in determining whether there will be a displacement of the fragments as a result of muscle pull. (See bottom insets in Plates 46 and 47.)

DISPLACEMENT IN UNILATERAL FRACTURE

(A) **Posterior Fragment (Ramus):** The ramus is pulled upward and forward by the elevator muscles if the line of fracture permits such displacement. Medial or lateral displacement is determined primarily by the direction of the blow and the line of fracture. In general, the masseter and internal pterygoid muscles tend to splint the fracture without displacement.

(B) **Anterior Fragment (Main Body):** The body of the mandible is depressed and rotated toward the injured side so that an open bite results on that side. This fragment is never greatly displaced and, unlike the posterior fragment, is easily controlled by occluding the teeth.

DISPLACEMENT IN BILATERAL FRACTURES

(A) **Posterior Fragments (Rami):** Both fragments are generally greatly displaced, since the restraining effect of the anterior fragment and the teeth is absent.

(B) **Anterior Fragment (Body of Mandible):** The displacement is unopposed and therefore downward and backward, resulting in a complete open bite (in both the anterior and the posterior region). The base of the tongue may be displaced backward, causing respiratory difficulties.

Reference: MAJOR, GLENN: Fractures of Jaws and Other Facial Bones. St. Louis: C. V. Mosby Co., 1943.

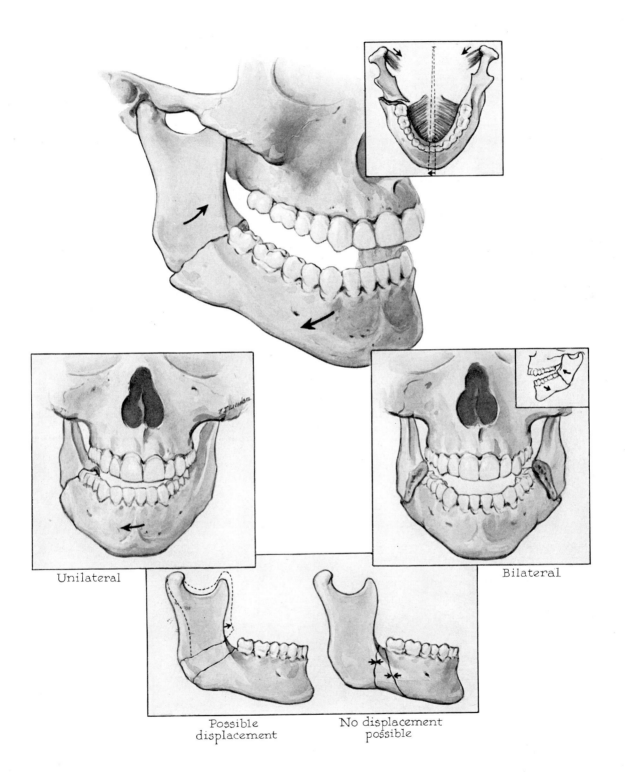

Unilateral

Bilateral

Possible
displacement

No displacement
possible

PLATE 46.

FRACTURES OF THE BODY OF THE MANDIBLE

FRACTURES through the body of the mandible are generally the result of direct blows. The line of fracture usually passes through the sockets of the adjacent teeth. The amount of displacement depends on:

1. The presence of opposing teeth, which tend to prevent upward displacement.
2. The angle of fracture, which may prevent or facilitate displacement.
3. The periosteum and surrounding soft tissue, which tend to limit displacement.

DISPLACEMENT IN UNILATERAL FRACTURE

(A) **Posterior Fragment:** If the portion of the body posteriorly from the line of fracture or the corresponding portion of the maxilla is edentulous, the fragment behaves like a fracture through the angle. (Plate 46.) If teeth are present in both the mandibular fragment and the corresponding maxillary portion, the upward displacement by the elevators is prevented by the occlusion of the teeth, unless there is also inward or outward displacement.

There is a marked tendency to medial displacement due to pull by the mylohyoid muscle.

(B) **Anterior Fragment:** The main body of the mandible is depressed and rotated toward the injured side so that an open bite results on that side. The position of the fracture is easily detected clinically by the difference in the occlusion of the posterior and anterior fragments.

DISPLACEMENT IN BILATERAL FRACTURES

(A) **Posterior Fragments:** Bilateral fractures through the body of the mandible generally occur in the mental regions. There is generally little displacement. If displacement does occur, it is easily controlled by occluding the teeth.

(B) **Anterior Fragment:** The small anterior fragment is pulled downward and, if the line of fracture permits, inward. The open bite between the anterior teeth is marked and characteristic.

Reference: FRY, W. K., et al.: Maxillofacial Injuries. Blackwell Scientific Publications, Oxford, 1943.

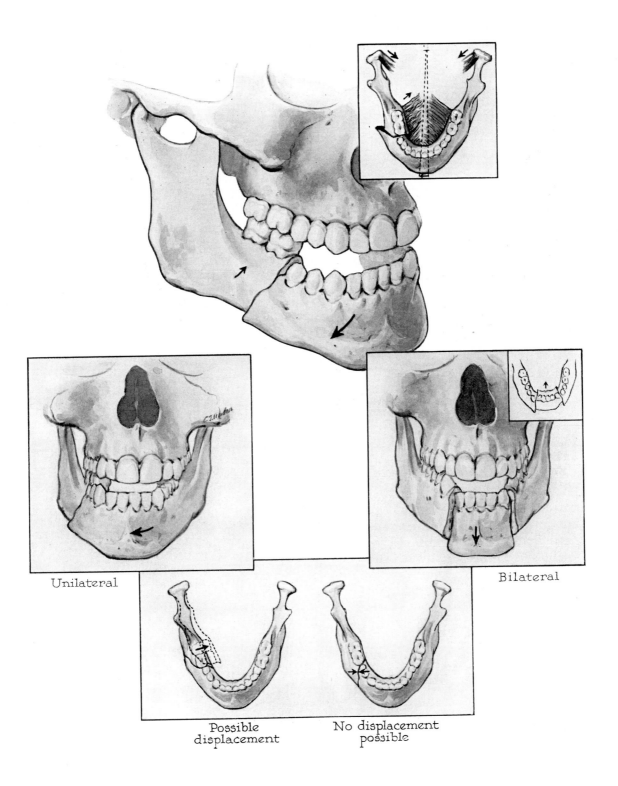

Unilateral

Bilateral

Possible
displacement

No displacement
possible

PLATE 47.

MULTIPLE FRACTURES OF THE MANDIBLE

DOUBLE or multiple fractures on the same side of the body of the mandible are generally the result of direct, smashing blows. The ramus fragment is rotated upward by the elevator muscles. The main fragment is depressed and rotated toward the injured side. The middle fragment is pulled downward and inward by the mylohyoid muscle.

Fractures of the body and the condylar neck or angle of the opposite side are generally the result of lateral blows on the mandible. These fractures are indirect. Each fragment is displaced as shown in Plates 44 to 47.

FRACTURE IN THE MIDLINE

When a fracture occurs in the midline of the mandible the fragments are seldom displaced since they have similar forces acting upon them. When displacement does result from the blow, the fragments are easily stabilized by ligating the teeth adjacent to the line of fracture. (See Horizontal Wiring, Plate 49.)

Reference: THOMA, K. H.: Traumatic Surgery of Jaws, Including First-Aid Treatment. St. Louis: C. V. Mosby Co., 1942.

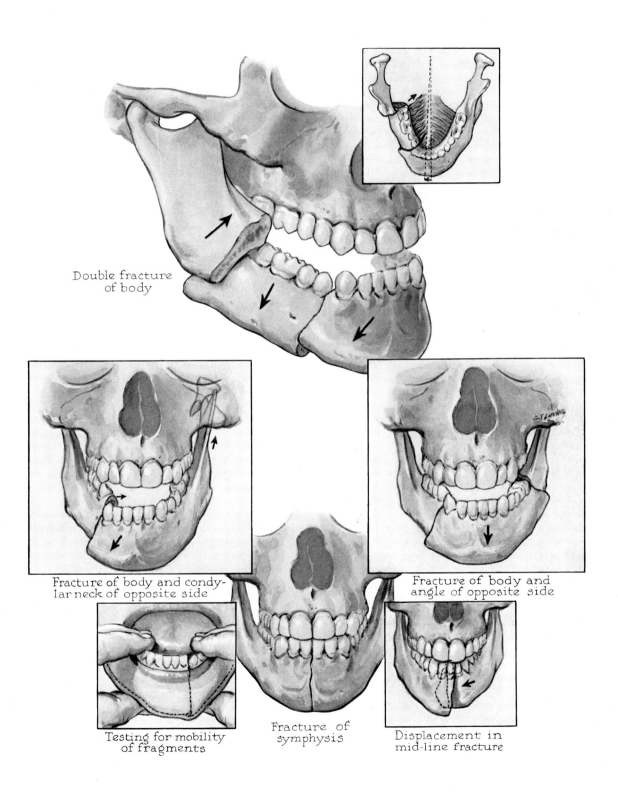

Double fracture
of body

Fracture of body and condylar neck of opposite side

Fracture of body and
angle of opposite side

Testing for mobility
of fragments

Fracture of
symphysis

Displacement in
mid-line fracture

PLATE 48.

TREATMENT OF MANDIBULAR FRACTURES

THE DENTIST is particularly qualified to cope with fractures of the jaws because of his specialized training in the occlusion of the teeth and in the construction of appliances for the jaws and teeth.

Every fracture should be reduced and immobilized at once. In case of displacement, examination of the occlusion will usually indicate the site of fracture. Bimanual manipulation will disclose abnormal mobility of the fragments and crepitus. Immediate reduction before trismus, pain and swelling have been allowed to develop, is relatively simple. If reduction is delayed, it may be necessary to use elastic traction or a general anesthetic to reduce the fracture. Emergency immobilization of the jaws in correct occlusion may be accomplished by different means. The head bandage is the simplest. Avoid the use of the Gibson bandage which forces the chin back and may cause gagging.

A more permanent fixation of the fracture is best accomplished by intermaxillary wiring, a few examples of which are shown. Reduction of fractures can be accomplished by the same means. Intramaxillary (single jaw) fixation by means of horizontal interdental wiring, metal arches (orthodontic arches), pins (Roger-Anderson) or splints (Gunning, Hammond) is frequently indicated, particularly in the armed forces where movement of the patient makes intermaxillary fixation undesirable because of the danger of vomiting. Various combinations are also possible, such as Colonel Stout's method of continuous wiring which combines the virtues of a number of methods. There is no universal or "best" method of fixation. The appliance must be made to fit the fracture—not vice versa.

Reference: WALDRON, C. W.: Fractures of the Mandible. The Journal-Lancet, Minneapolis, 62:228-240, June 1942.

TREATMENT OF MANDIBULAR FRACTURES

IMMEDIATE REDUCTION AND IMMOBILIZATION

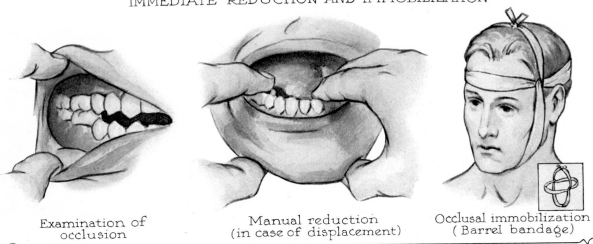

Examination of
occlusion

Manual reduction
(in case of displacement)

Occlusal immobilization
(Barrel bandage)

INTERMAXILLARY REDUCTION AND FIXATION

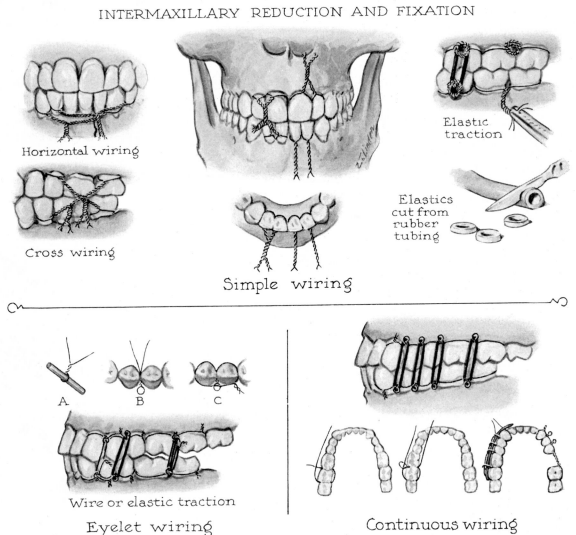

Horizontal wiring

Cross wiring

Simple wiring

Elastic
traction

Elastics
cut from
rubber
tubing

A   B   C

Wire or elastic traction

Eyelet wiring

Continuous wiring

PLATE 49.